PLASMA FRACTIONATION AND BLOOD TRANSFUSION

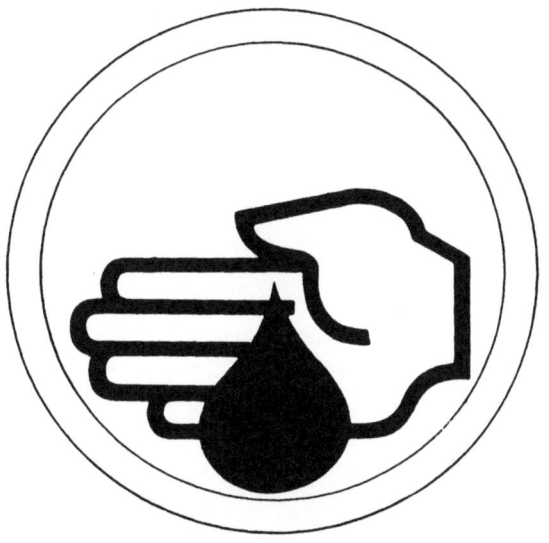

DEVELOPMENTS IN HEMATOLOGY AND IMMUNOLOGY

Lijnen, H.R., Collen, D. and Verstraete, M., eds: Synthetic Substrates in Clinical Blood Coagulation Assays. 1980. ISBN 90-247-2409-0

Smit Sibinga, C.Th., Das, P.C. and Forfar, J.O., eds: Paediatrics and Blood Transfusion. 1982. ISBN 90-247-2619-0

Fabris, N., ed: Immunology and Ageing. 1982. ISBN 90-247-2640-9

Hornstra, G.: Dietary Fats, Prostanoids and Arterial Thrombosis. 1982. ISBN 90-247-2667-0

Smit Sibinga, C.Th., Das, P.C. and Loghem, van J.J., eds: Blood Transfusion and Problems of Bleeding. 1982. ISBN 90-247-3058-9

Dormandy, J., ed: Red Cell Deformability and Filterability. 1983. ISBN 0-89838-578-4

Smit Sibinga, C.Th., Das, P.C. and Taswell, H.F., eds: Quality Assurance in Blood Banking and Its Clinical Impact. 1984. ISBN 0-89838-618-7

Besselaar, A.M.H.P. van den, Gralnick, H.R. and Lewis, S.M., eds: Thromboplastin Calibration and Oral Anticoagulant Control. 1984. ISBN 0-89838-637-3

Fondu, P. and Thijs, O., eds: Haemostatic Failure in Liver Disease. 1984. ISBN 0-89838-640-3

Smit Sibinga, C.Th., Das, P.C. and Opelz, G., eds: Transplantation and Blood Transfusion. 1984. ISBN 0-89838-686-1

Schmid-Schönbein, H., Wurzinger, L.J. and Zimmerman, R.E., eds: Enzyme Activation in Blood-Perfused Artificial Organs. 1985. ISBN 0-89838-704-3

Dormandy, J., ed: Blood Filtration and Blood Cell Deformability. 1985. ISBN 0-89838-714-0

Smit Sibinga, C.Th., Das, P.C. and Seidl, S., eds: Plasma Fractionation and Blood Transfusion. 1985. ISBN 0-89838-761-2

Plasma Fractionation and Blood Transfusion

Proceedings of the Ninth Annual Symposium on Blood Transfusion, Groningen, 1984, organized by the Red Cross Blood Bank Groningen-Drenthe

edited by

C.Th. SMIT SIBINGA and P.C. DAS

Red Cross Blood Bank Groningen-Drenthe
The Netherlands

S. SEIDL

Red Cross Blood Transfusion Service Hessen
Frankfurt am Main
F.R.G.

1985 **MARTINUS NIJHOFF PUBLISHERS**
a member of the KLUWER ACADEMIC PUBLISHERS GROUP
BOSTON / DORDRECHT / LANCASTER

Distributors

for the United States and Canada: Kluwer Academic Publishers, 190 Old Derby Street, Hingham, MA 02043, USA
for the UK and Ireland: Kluwer Academic Publishers, MTP Press Limited, Falcon House, Queen Square, Lancaster LA1 1RN, UK
for all other countries: Kluwer Academic Publishers Group, Distribution Center, P.O. Box 322, 3300 AH Dordrecht, The Netherlands

Library of Congress Cataloging in Publication Data

ISBN-13: 978-1-4612-9644-7   e-ISBN-13: 978-1-4613-2631-1
DOI: 10.1007/978-1-4613-2631-1

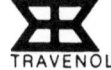

Acknowledgement

This publication has been made possible through the support of Travenol, which is gratefully acknowledged.

CONTENTS

MODERATORS

S. Seidl (chairman)	— Red Cross Blood Transfusion Service Hessen Frankfurt am Main, FRG
H.G.J. Brummelhuis	— Central Laboratory of the Blood Transfusion Amsterdam, NL
R.A. Coutinho	— Municipal Health Service Amsterdam, Amsterdam, NL
H.H. Gunson	— National Blood Transfusion Service, Manchester, UK
J. Over	— Central Laboratory of the Blood Transfusion Amsterdam, NL
F. Peetoom	— American Red Cross Blood Services Portland, OR, USA
J.K. Smith	— Plasma Fractionation Laboratory, Oxford, UK
C.Th. Smit Sibinga	— Red Cross Blood Bank Groningen-Drenthe Groningen, NL

SPEAKERS

J.B. Bussel	— The New York Hospital-Cornell Medical Center New York, NY, USA
J. Curling	— Pharmacia Fine Chemicals, Uppsala, S
P.R. Foster	— Scottish National Blood Transfusion Service Edinburgh, UK
R.J. Gerety	— Office of Biologics Research and Review Bethesda, MD, USA
J. Goudsmit	— University of Amsterdam, Amsterdam, NL
S. Iwarson	— University of Göteborg, Göteborg, S
J.M. Jason	— Center for Infectious Diseases, Atlanta, GA, USA
W.C. Lake	— Travenol Laboratories Inc. Deerfield, IL, USA
S.H. Middleton	— Speywood Laboratories Ltd, Wexham, UK
I.M. Nilsson	— Allmänna Sjukhuset, Malmö, S
U.E. Nydegger	— Central Laboratory of the Swiss Blood Transfusion Service, Bern, CH
C.V. Prowse	— Edinburgh and South-East Scotland Regional Blood Transfusion Service Edinburgh, UK
E.L. Snyder	— Yale University, New Haven, CT, USA

PREPARED DISCUSSANTS

P.C. Das	— Red Cross Bloodbank Groningen-Drenthe, Groningen, NL
A.D. Friesen	— The Winnipeg Rh Institute Inc., Winnipeg, C
F. Haskó	— National Institute of Haematology and Blood Transfusion, Budapest, H
P.B.A. Kernoff	— Royal Free Hospital, London, UK
W. Stephan	— Biotest Pharma GmbH, Frankfurt, FRG

FOREWORD

Plasma fractionation and blood transfusion are inherently linked. Blood-bankers need to have a sincere interest in fractionation and purification techniques in order to understand the need for carefully controlled source material collection and initial processing. Developments point to a shift in technology, implementation and application of plasma fractions to be produced, such that early anticipation from both bloodbankers and fractionators in a joint interest and effort are needed.

As usual there is good news and bad news. We are referring in that respect to the exciting presentation about the future of bloodbanking. Although the blood donor still plays a major role in bloodbanking, new technologies could terminate the conventional blood transfusion service in the next 20-40 years. Sooner or later DNA technology will play an important role in bloodbanking and bloodbankers will have to deal with cultivated red cells as a replacement of our donor blood. Several fractionation techniques like column chromatography, controlled pore glass chromatography, heparin double cold precipitation technology and polyelectrolite fractionation are available, which may result in better yields for some of the plasma proteins. These techniques are likely to replace in part the old Cohn fractionation in the near future.

For logistic reasons it should be reemphasized that sufficient FVIII yield can be obtained from blood which has been stored for 18 hours. However, it should also be kept in mind that significantly better yields are achieved by fast freezing immediately following collection, the use of CPDA anticoagulant or plasmapheresis by machines. Additionally, the yield may be influenced by the storage technique. It seems also likely to further increase the FVIII yield by applying special absorption techniques and the use of heparin.

An important point of discussion at present is whether a centralized fractionation is always advantageous. It is our feeling that there are certainly advantages when some of the plasma proteins, FVIII for instance, are prepared in regional centres. However, some other plasma proteins still do require a more centralized approach. The solution for the future might be a marriage of both systems.

Besides achievements of higher yields and better purities through newly developed fractionation techniques, maintenance of function is a major safety concern in plasma separation. To reduce the transmission of infectious agents, new screening procedures are likely to be introduced in the near future. For instance, reverse transcriptase as a test to detect carriers of non A non B might be around the corner. For hepatitis B effective screening procedures are already available as well as vaccines. This might eradicate hepatitis B following transfusion. But we are still dealing with products potentially contaminated with infectious viruses. Methods to inactivate, neutralize or remove these agents are outlined, giving preference to inactivation techniques.

First results of ongoing studies are reported regarding the detectability of HTLV-III antibodies among various groups. Recipients of FVIII demonstrated the highest percentage in relation to the amount of FVIII given to these patients. Various recent studies showed efficacy of heat treatment to inactivate HTLV-III. Heat treatment of freeze-dried preparations is shown as effective as heat treatment of wet preparations. During the panel discussions the question of routine screening of blood donors has been extensively covered. Prospective studies are ongoing in the United States and commercial tests on ELISA basis are about to be licensed. However, a number of questions related to HTLV infection and AIDS needs full attention in the near future. What is the natural history of the disease? What is the meaning of anti-HTLV-III positivity?

The clinical aspects of some important plasma derivatives are discussed. FVIII concentrates of various manufacturers showed marked differences in the FVIII related antigen concentration. Of clinical importance, however, is the observation that the half-life of heat treated and non heat treated FVIII preparations are similar. Although the question of standardisation of FVIII assay has been raised, the difficulties are clearly demonstrated.

Polyelectrolite fractionated porcine FVIII preparations are obtained with an extremely high purity and a reduced reactivity with most inhibitors. These preparations are likely to provide a good alternative in the treatment of inhibitor patients.

The role of fibronectin is still an open question. Clinical studies showed that lower levels of fibronectin were only seen consistently in critically ill patients, although there is a discrepancy between immuno and bio-assays of fibronectin. For the time being there is no specific patient group to be recommended for fibronectin treatment. The possible indications for intravenous immunoglobulins are outlined. There are two types of diseases where IVIgG has been shown to be a useful therapy: Antibody deficiency and autoimmune diseases. IVIgG preparations can be considered as safe products specifically with respect to transmission of hepatitis and HTLV-III.

These proceedings of the 9th international symposium on blood transfusion, organised by the Red Cross Blood Bank Groningen-Drenthe, provide a comprehensive overview of the state of the art in plasma fractionation, giving at the same time a challenging perspective for the future in bloodbanking.

C.Th. Smit Sibinga
P.C. Das
S. Seidl   editors

OPENING ADDRESS

G.E. Schuth, president executive board, Red Cross Blood Bank
Groningen-Drenthe

With pleasure I accepted the invitation to open this symposium. This
9th meeting organized by the Red Cross Blood Bank Groningen-Drenthe,
is on plasma fractionation and blood transfusion.
Over the last 3 decades, many developments in surgery and medicine
have relied heavily on voluntary blood donations which have continued
to sustain this progress, saved many lives and reduced much suffering.
The concept of component therapy, where blood products are separated
into effective clinical components, has been exciting. In a real sense
this progress has become a breathtakingly exciting with plasma fractionation, not only new therapeutic products have emerged but the purity
of others has increased. Yet these advances have generated problems
of their own, mostly related to the quality and quantity aspects: larger
pool sizes tend to increase loss during fractionation, and also enhance
potential hazards for disease transmission. Some of these problems have
been attacked successfully, for instance, by attempting alternative
fractionation methods, and by introducing the use of small pools. The
self sufficiency of the community relating to plasma components is a
strongly felt issue; a nation's clinical requirement and its own plasma
supply are not always subjected to an unbiased equation. However, all
these factors are closely interlocked with the rapidly changing scientific
developments, and a small percentage production increase could make
a community self-surplus instead of undertaking expensive investment
for collecting extra plasma. Before making such investments it ought
to be recognised that the traditional activities in a blood bank and
transfusion service might undergo significant changes. This is due
partly to the changes occurring in patients management, but mostly
to the rapidly advancing biotechnology, promising safer and purer
products. Thus, the future world of blood transfusion is full of
excitement, not least for the voluntary blood donors whose precious
gift and its optimal use remain pre-eminant today.
On behalf of the Executive Committee of the Red Cross Blood Bank
Groningen-Drenthe and the organizers, I have great pleasure in
declaring this meeting open. The programme looks excellent, the chairman and moderators are internationally known, and the speakers are
experts. I wish you a successful meeting, and hand over to the
chairman Professor Seidl.

I. Source material

THE FUTURE BLOOD SUPPLY SYSTEM IN THE USA: A PROGNOSIS

F. Peetoom and S.M. Gaynor

MAJOR FACTORS WHICH WILL DETERMINE THE FUTURE NEEDS FOR BLOOD SERVICES IN THE USA

1. Demographic developments are directly tied to health care needs and, therefore, to blood needs. Major national demographic determinants are population growth, including factors such as birth, immigration and life expectancy rates, and population age distribution. At the regional level, developments in migration and ethnic distribution patterns are of additional importance. The movement of the 'baby boom' through the 25- to 40-year age bracket should initially improve the blood-giving segment of the eligible population. However, 20 to 30 years from now, the front runners of the 'baby boom' will begin to enter, in significant numbers, the high blood-using age period. The prediction is that this will result in a change in the blood donor to blood recipient ratio from 8 to 1 in the 70's to 3 to 1 in 2025. This particular demographic evolution is probably the single most important one affecting blood supply and needs early in the 21st century.

2. Medical practices, on the one hand, will look for more specific targeting of therapy and treatment, in order to reduce unwanted, transfusion requiring side-effects, such as general bone marrow suppression due to various chemotherapies. If this can be accomplished by means of e.g. clinically applied immunological principles, a considerable reduction in demand for several types of blood products may be anticipated. On the other hand, historically, new uses of blood and blood products have consistently shown an upward trend. A similar trend in the future can be expected, and can be anticipated as a continuing driving force in the growing demand for blood.

3. Economic developments are now effectively putting a brake on health care expenditures in the USA. It is anticipated that future blood demands will be affected by currently evolving reimbursement policies, particularly in those situations where blood might be prescribed as a 'tonic' rather than as a life-saving or life-sustaining product. This influence is applauded by many, in that it might serve as an added opportunity to educate practicing physicians in realistic hemotherapy. This opportunity might help to resolve the much debated issue of demand versus true need for blood.

4. Socio-political developments may become increasingly influenced by the needs of a growing number of older people. This could well mean that rather than fewer federal and state dollars for health care of the elderly, there would be considerable political pressure from the aging for more support in the future. Some futuristic views hold that social attitudes will deteriorate towards a more self-centered state, resulting in a more defensive, self-protective posture. This would be the consequence of a pressured, high performance demanding society under

4

conditions of depersonalized relationships. Such a development would manifest itself in decreased sensitivity to others' needs, and require increased investments for blood donor recruitment to be successful.

The above are just some examples of probable or possible developments that will affect blood needs and blood supply conditions in the USA in times to come. Next, we will present a scenario of how the future needs for blood are going to be met.

PROGNOSIS OF FUTURE BLOOD SERVICE DELIVERY

The 'Blood Service Delivery Box' illustrates our hypothesis of the evolution of the supply mechanisms in the next 50 years (fig. 1).
  The Classical or Traditional Supply System (1), as we currently know it, illustrated in Time Level 1, will continue to function for many more years, meeting increasing demands for blood products with increasing difficulty. Factors which will cause such difficulty include the earlier described demographic development (increasing users vs. decreasing donors), changing donor attitudes, and growing doubts about the social and safety aspects of paid plasma donors and the rising cost of the Classical System. The resulting, visible distress symptoms become the driving force behind accelerated attempts in the recombinant DNA industry to produce specific plasma proteins such as albumin, AHF, erythropoetin, antithrombin, and others, in increasing variety and quantity. These incentives will not only come from the national market but from international markets as well.

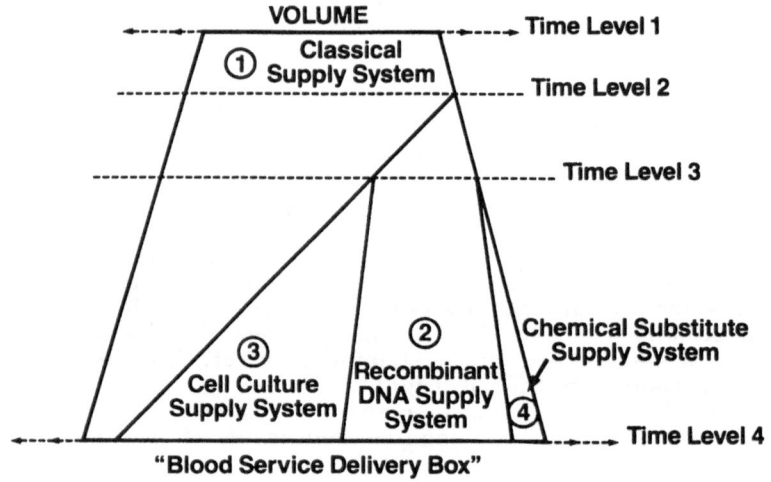

"Blood Service Delivery Box"
1. Whole Blood Collections, Plasma- and Cytapheresis
2. Growing Number of Specialized Plasma Proteins: Biological Plasma Substitutes
Cell Culture "Co-Factors"
3. Red Cells, Platelets, Specialized White Blood Cells
4. Chemically-Produced Substitutes for a Limited Number of Blood Elements/Factors

Figure 1. Prognosis of future blood service delivery.

The initiation of recombinant plasma protein supply, as shown in Time Level 2, will significantly affect the value of plasma provided through the classical supply system. The number of different products which will have to be met from this historical plasma source will be gradually reduced. Because of ongoing concerns of safety, the clinical use of human-derived biologicals will be avoided when possible. This development will greatly reduce the economic incentives for the commercial plasmapheresis industry. Further, the loss of economic value of plasma will add to the charges for cellular components produced in the whole blood procurement system. In other words, at this point, the traditional supply system will begin to suffer from a rapidly growing number of untreatable dilemmas.

We are now in Time Level 3. The recombinant DNA process will begin to produce and/or scale up existing production of those regulating substances and co-factors that have been recognized as essential. Both, in the in vivo and in vitro propagation and differentiation of the three major blood cell lines. The industrial, large scale production of transfusable blood cells is critically dependent on the recombinant DNA industry. No other mechanism or source can provide the quantities of ingredients necessary for the industrial conversion of the classical blood-cell supply system, although some chemically produced co-factors will substitute for biological originals. The introduction of industrial methods for the provision of cellular blood components, even if only one component is initially available, will further deteriorate the economic viability of the classical supply system and seriously erode its prospects of long term survival.

There will be growing expectations of this new and competitive, free enterprise industrial supply system that not only can eliminate disease from blood products, but can provide them at lower cost. Eventually, the industrial parts of the blood service delivery complex will greatly dominate the largest segment of the hemotherapy market, leaving a decreasing number of very expensive unique compatibility issues to be addressed and resolved by a shrinking number of classical suppliers.

The provision of blood products through in vitro technology will have a considerable impact on the organizational elements in the classical blood service delivery system. Some of the larger blood centers may become directly involved in the application of these new technologies that will lead to the replacement of a majority of donor-derived transfusable blood products. Because of the associated, high development and capital investment costs, pooling of resources would seem the necessary mechanism for non-profit blood banking organizations to compete, or to be a partner with industry in this field. The industrial component, which emerges as the alternate provider, will most probably consist of partnerships among current 'high-tech' companies, plasma fractionators and/or microbial vaccine manufacturers. It appears that the combined technologies of these three industries would serve as the foundation for large scale production development.

The great majority of traditional blood banks will face a substantial decline in blood collection and blood processing volume (fig. 2). For the smaller volume centres, which do not have the option of offering an expanded services package, this will mean a choice between integration in a larger regional blood service system (in order to benefit from resource sharing, and to reduce overhead costs), or going out of business. Other than on simple economics, the survival of blood banks during the transformation period will depend on the evolution of the level of medical care in the institutions they serve. Advanced medical care will tend to generate new and special demands which will require blood bank service

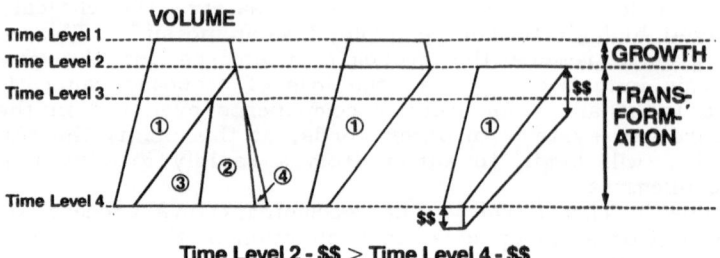

Figure 2. Growth and transformation of classical supply system.

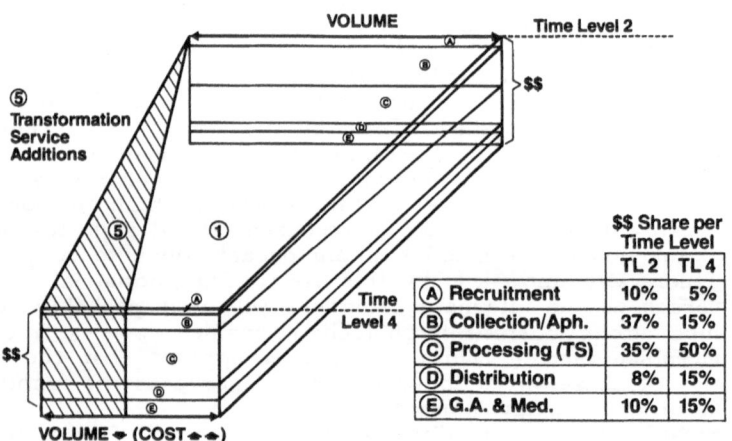

Figure 3.

additions and supply logistics that may serve as economical and political keys to continued operation.

Let us, now, discuss more specifically the impact of the in vitro blood supply system on the five major functions of the traditional blood bank or centre. These functions are: donor recruitment, blood collection and hemapheresis, blood processing and technical services, product management and distribution, general administration and medical services (fig. 3).

1. Donor recruitment: The red cell product, prepared in vitro, will be close to universal donor group and type, in that it will be group O and negative for the majority of immunogenic blood types. However, this will not universally prevent recipient sensitization and, since red cell antibody stimulation will also continue to occur through non-transfusion related routes, access to compatible, rare donor blood will remain a requirement. This will necessitate a rare donor inventory which can only be established through extensive testing of many donors. In addition, the need for an increasingly larger group of HLA and DR typed donors for HLA-matched blood product transfusion and for transplantation purposes, respectively, makes a considerably reduced donor recruitment department still an essential element in the transformation phase. If tissue banking would become an integral part of blood centre activities, tissue procurement and organ donor recruitment might slow down the decline of this blood centre function.

2. Blood collection and hemapheresis: The function responsible for collection of random donor blood for the preparation of transfusable products will become quite insignificant, both, in comparison to its current size and as a department in the transformation-period blood services organization. One of its roles will be to collect blood specimens for testing of potential, volunteer donors. This will permit the development of a general back-up donor file, the identification of rare donors and the needed inventory of donors typed for HLA and other cellular antigen systems (DR, Pl, NA). Based on demand for specifically matched blood components, as well as for therapeutic services, hemapheresis will continue to be a growing function throughout the transformation period.

3. Blood processing and technical services: This function will grow in relative and absolute size throughout the transformation period, despite a substantial decline in traditional activities. Comprehensive and expanded testing of the required inventory of potential donors will contribute to a predictable growth in further specialized, technical equipment and facilities to be used for this purpose. Increases in demand for hemapheresis products are also paralleled by expanded compatibility testing and processing capabilities which presently are in early stages of development. Blood centres in the appropriate medical markets may assume a centralized role in tissue procurement, processing, storage and distribution. In addition, several new technical-services and reference-services opportunities are now emerging, and more ar expected to be conceived in the future. In our opinion, the technical services functions of blood centres will benefit from the prevailing condition of limited growth in health care dollars, in that it permits centralized support of highly specialized nature to meet regional needs in a most proficient and most economical manner.

4. Product management and distribution: Because of their perishable nature, the growing supply of blood products from industrial sources

will still require an effective and efficient inventory management and distribution system, even with improved storage and dating. It seems likely that the traditional blood supply network will turn out to be the ideal support system. The prediction, then, is that this regional blood centre function will gain in absolute and relative size because of an overall increase in transfusion activities, and also, due to the addition of new products.

5.   General administration and medical services: Because of the ongoing upgrading of management information systems to serve overall administrative and operational management of the increasingly complex blood centre activities, the administrative function will continue to demand relatively large budget allocations. Medical services provided by the blood centre will tend to increase because of their favorable cost-effective position in several hematological services areas.

SUMMARY

We would like to conclude that the role of blood centres that survive the transformation period of the blood supply system evolution will remain crucial to the future health care system in the USA. Compared to the original, first-generation functions, performed by blood banks 30 years ago, and relative to the much expanded, second-generation blood services provided today, there are positive indications that many of our current blood centres will have the opportunity to face the challenge of third-generation blood service demands of a new future.

PLASMA SUPPLY
NATIONAL AND INTERNATIONAL LOGISTICS, WHOLE BLOOD VERSUS
PLASMAPHERESIS

H.H. Gunson

INTRODUCTION

There has been a great deal of discussion about the international supply
of plasma during recent years. In 1975, the World Health Assembly urged
member states to 'promote the development of national blood services
based on voluntary non-remunerated donation of blood ...' Subsequently
the International Society of Blood Transfusion, together with the League
of Red Cross Societies prepared a Code of Ethics on Blood Donation and
Transfusion which embodied the principle detailed above.

It has been estimated (1), that of the seven million litres plasma fractionated annually, more than 80 per cent is derived from commercial
plasmapheresis. There is a question which must be asked: is it feasible
for countries to become self-sufficient with respect to plasma supply? In
this presentation an attempt will be made to analyse this problem and
the possibilities of the methods available to achieve this aim will be discussed. It should be stressed that any opinions given in the paper are
those of the author and should not be interpreted as the policy of a
government or other body.

PLASMA REQUIREMENTS

Many products can be purified from plasma but there are two broad
groups of products which must be considered when calculating the requirements for plasma self-sufficiency, viz.: those products derived
from normal human plasma and those from hyperimmune antibody containing plasma.

The demand for the latter has been increasing over the past few
years concurrently with the more frequent use of chemotherapy which
suppresses the immune response. In general the plasma requirement for
these preparations does not pose the logistic problems caused by the
production of normal human plasma since it can be obtained from relatively fewer donors by plasmapheresis. Use of immunoglobulins varies
widely and it is not possible to estimate accurately the plasma requirement. Whilst this aspect of self-sufficiency cannot be ignored, I propose
to concentrate below on the supply of normal human plasma.

Three major classes of products are derived from normal human
plasma, viz.: coagulation factors, normal immunoglobulin and albumin.
Whilst the development of intravenous immunoglobulin will undoubtedly
lead to an increased use of this product, it is the requirement for
factor VIII concentrates and albumin preparations which will determine
the quantity of plasma required for the national attainment of self-sufficiency in blood products, since if demand for these products can be
satisfied sufficient plasma will be available for the preparation of other
products.

The term 'driving force', used to indicate the particular product which relates to the volume of plasma required has been commonly used. In many countries it is the need for factor VIII concentrates which has provided this driving force, whilst in others, notably in Japan, the use of albumin predominates. The ISBT Working Party on Socio-Economic Aspects of Blood Transfusion (1983) concluded that the term 'driving force' was counter-productive and the main effort should be directed towards a nationally managed balanced blood supply for all clinical needs (2). Nevertheless, it has been the 'driving force' for the collection of red cells in optimum quantities, arguably the first priority in any national blood program, which has contributed to the present unsatisfactory international situation with respect to plasma supply. It is recognised that approximately 50,000 donors per million of the population will satisfy red cell needs. Removal of 200-225 ml plasma from 60 percent of the donations collected will yield 6000-6750 litres plasma per million of the population. With the use of optimal additive solutions when 250-280 ml plasma can be removed from each whole blood donation 7500-8400 litres plasma per million of the population can be obtained.

REQUIREMENT OF PLASMA FOR FACTOR VIII CONCENTRATES

It is pertinent to examine the plasma needs, particularly for factor VIII concentrates since there has been a changing pattern in the treatment of patients suffering from hemophilia A during the past decade, in particular with home therapy to provide early treatment of bleeding episodes and the increasing use of prophylactic substitution therapy (3). The use of factor VIII concentrates has been increasing annually and this can be illustrated by the statistics for the United Kingdom where 25 million units (approximately 0.4 units per head of the population) was used in 1975 compared with an estimated total of 75 million units (1.25 units per head) in 1983. There is evidence that this total is insufficient and an estimate of 2 units per head of the population is now generally recognised. Even this may be an underestimate and several workers in the field are predicting a rise to 2.5 or even 2.75 units factor VIII per head of the population (Cash, personal communication).

There are many variables involved in cryoprecipitation and in order to obtain the minimum supply of plasma it is important to take advantage of as many of these which enhance the yield of factor VIII. However, where blood donations are being collected from randomly selected donors by mobile collection teams operating at a distance from their blood transfusion centres, this may be difficult. These factors include the freezing of plasma to lower than -30°C within two hours of collection (4) the selection of donors of group A or AB (5) or the use of 1-desamino-8-D-arginine (DDAVP) which significantly increases factor VIII levels in plasma, best introduced by the intranasal route one hour before donation to minimise side effects (6). Also, it must be remembered that in the scaling-up of fractionation processes it may not be possible to take advantage of procedures which increase the yield of factor VIII from the source plasma pool. Such procedures include rapid thaw (4), agitation (7), or removal of residual plasma by syphoning (8), although with respect to the latter Foster et al. (9) by enhancing thawing by using thin films with large surface areas have shown experimentally that a significant increase in factor VIII yield can be obtained. The use of heparinized plasma may also be an important factor (10) and the value of this product in large scale fractionation merits further investigation. A further factor which has to be taken into account is that coagulation factor concentrates are known to transmit diseases; although the transmission of AIDS has received much publicity recently it is the transmission of non-A non-B hepatitis which, arguably, poses the greater problem. The need for concentrates which will lessen these risks is clear. However, methods which have been applied to remove viruses compromise the yield of coagulation factor activity and unless this can be compensated for by an initial higher yield prior to treatment, it will inevitably mean that a greater volume of plasma will be required to achieve self-sufficiency.

In calculating the volume of plasma required to satisfy the factor VIII concentrate need, it has been assumed that for intermediate concentrate a net yield of 225 IU per litre of starting plasma can be achieved. For 2 million units per million of the population per year, this will required 9,600 litres per million of the population. If freeze-dried cryoprecipitate is the basic product used, at a yield of 300 IU per litre plasma, 8000 litres of plasma per year will be needed. In both instances it has been assumed that a supplement of high purity concentrate, at a yield of 150 IU per litre plasma, will be necessary for selected patients. Britten (11) has also arrived at essentially similar conclusions. If the requirement for factor VIII concentrates exceeds the estimate of 2 million units per million of the population, then the plasma requirement will be increased proportionately.

MEANS OF OBTAINING PLASMA

It is clear from the above that the separation of plasma leaving the red cells untreated as a concentrate suspended in residual plasma will not allow the collection of plasma for what are now being regarded as minimum requirements for factor VIII concentrates. Also, it should be remembered that red cell sufficiency may not reach 50,000 per million inhabitants, particularly when a shelf-life of 35 days is now common practice. It is significant in those countries where the policy of obtaining source plasma from whole blood donations with red cell concentrates as the by-product has been adopted, blood collection has had to be increased above 50,000 per million inhabitants and this has led to a wastage of the cells or disposal of the red cell concentrates to countries where a shortage exists. One can argue the ethics of discarding red cells from a donor and there are donors who would accept that whilst their donation is not being used to total effect, their contribution to the national program is still worthwhile and justified. On the other hand, sending the surplus red cell concentrates to another country may have the effect of discouraging that country to develop a self-sufficiency in plasma particularly if this results in their red cell requirement being fulfilled.

Making use of additive solutions could possibly satisfy plasma requirements for factor VIII but would preclude the modest purification of factor VIII preparations. Also it must be remembered that the use of single donations of fresh plasma increases when a large number of red cells in additive solutions are used. The hemophilia treatment would have to be based upon freeze-dried cryoprecipitate. It may be difficult in some countries to achieve the required standards put forward by national regulatory authorities when this product is manufactured, particularly if it is prepared from small plasma pools. Nevertheless, the use of optimal additive solutions represents a significant advance in collecting the maximum quantity of plasma from a donation of whole blood and can provide the basis of a national program.

Plasmapheresis has, for many years, been the principle procedure for the collection of plasma by commercial organisations and has been used also by certain national programs with some success. Plasmapheresis has both advantages and disadvantages. Advantages include: (i) the smaller number of donors required to obtain a given quantity of plasma since approximately 500 ml can be obtained at a single procedure, and with the recognised limit of 15 litres plasma per year a donor can undergo 30 procedures each years; (ii) donors can be selected for blood group with a predominence given to those of group A and AB; (iii) with regular attendance at a plasmapheresis centre DDAVP could be used to raise factor VIII levels in the plasma, although the long-term effects of such treatment requires careful assessment; (iv) plasma can be rapidly frozen after collection and (v) with the more recent techniques of filtration plasmapheresis it is possible to obtain almost cell-free plasma. This may carry advantages with respect to the quality of factor VIII preparations and also increase the yield, factors which are being studied at present. Disadvantages include: (i) the time taken for donation which with the manual procedure is 1-1½ hours and maybe a disincentive to donors although the more recent machines have reduced this time to approximately 35 minutes which may prove more acceptable; (ii) again with manual systems the return of the wrong red cells to the donor is a potential danger also eliminated by the machine procedure, and (iii) cost of the plasma compared with that obtained as a by-product of the preparation of red cells. The cost-factor, however, must be considered carefully since in recent years the cost of machines for plasmapheresis and the disposables they use have been reducing and there is substance in the argument that plasma is only more cost-effective when collected from donations of whole blood provided there is a use for the red cells. When the residual red cells are discarded, the full cost of collecting the donation in addition to the costs of plasma separation must be added to the cost of plasma.

The author's view is that plasma should be separated from donations of whole blood, using optimal additive solutions where possible, until the red cell requirement has been reached, thereafter plasmapheresis is the procedure of choice.

ALBUMIN PREPARATIONS

The collection of 8000-9600 litres plasma to provide self-sufficiency in factor VIII concentrates will, following sequential fractionation, yield between 185 and 220 kg albumin per million of the population. This approximates with the average assessment of albumin requirement made in 1978 by a study group of the Council of Europe (12). The use of albumin preparations varies widely throughout the world as has been noted previously and such quantities would not be sufficient in certain countries if present usage levels were to continue. However, in any national self-sufficiency program for plasma collection there will be surpluses of certain products and this will likely include albumin in a number of countries. By international co-operation export of albumin products from countries where the usage is low is a means for solving the international demand. Finally, it is apparent that the first priority of any country is to achieve self-sufficiency in red cells. Once that has been attained, attention should be given to the collection of sufficient plasma in order to obtain self-sufficiency in fractionated blood products. The contribution which commercial organisations can make towards this effort should be carefully considered. It is not the standard of production facilities for which industry can be criticized, but their source of plasma which is derived from remunerated donors. Even if a country achieves self-sufficiency in plasma supply it may not be cost-effective to build a fractionation plant and co-operation with industry may be a logical way in which to further the interests of that country. Also, world-wide distribution of surplus products could well be undertaken by commercial organisations, to the benefit of many countries. One cannot expect such companies to operate without profit, otherwise they would become non-viable.

It is not yet known what the effect will be on this international logistical problem from the production of certain blood products by genetic engineering and in this, industry will have a large part to play. One cannot isolate one product, e.g. factor VIII without there being a considerable effect on others which continue to be derived from plasma. I suspect that plasma will be required throughout the world for the foreseeable future to come and whilst the principles of the World Health Assembly, stated at the beginning of this paper, should be given the highest priority by National Health Authorities and other bodies committed to the organisation of blood services, co-operation with industry under the terms which I have outlined could ultimately be beneficial.

REFERENCES

1. Britten AFH. The solution to adequate plasma supplies. Abstracts of the 18th Congress of the International Society of Blood Transfusion. S. Karger, Basel 1984:16-7.
2. Socio-economic aspects of blood transfusion. Moore BPL, Beal RW eds. Vox Sang 1984;46 (suppl. 1).
3. Preparation and use of coagulation factors VIII and IX for transfusion. European Health Committee, Council of Europe, Strasbourg, 1980.
4. Wensley RT, Snape TS. Preparation of improved cryoprecipitated Factor VIII concentrate: A controlled study of three variables affecting the yield. Vox Sang 1980;38:222-8.
5. Preston AE, Barr A. The plasma concentration of factor VIII in the normal population. II The effects of age, sex and blood group. Brit J Haemat 1964;10:238-45.
6. Mikaelson M, Nilsson IM, Villardt H, Wiechel B. Factor VIII concentrate prepared from blood donors stimulated with intranasal DDAVP. Transfusion 1982;22:229-33.
7. Margolis J. Improvements in production of anti-haemophilic factor (VIII) concentrates. Proceedings of XIth Congress of World Federation of Hemophilia 1976:223.
8. Mason EC. Thaw-syphon technique for the production of cryoprecipitate concentrate of factor VIII. Lancet 1978;ii:15-7.
9. Foster PR, Dickson AJ, McQuillan TA, Dickson IH, Keddie S, Watt J. Control of large-scale plasma thawing for recovery of cryoprecipitated Factor VIII. Vox Sang 1982;42:180-9.
10. Rock GA, Cruikshank WH, Thackabery ES, Palmer DS. Improved yields of Factor VIII from heparinized plasma. Vox Sang 1979;36:294-300.
11. Britten AFH. Plasma procurement and fractionation: A world-wide review. In: Plasma products: Use and management. Kolins J, Britten AFH, Silvergleid AJ, eds. American Association of Blood Banks, Arlington 1982:1-22.

12. Indications for the use of albumin, plasma protein solutions and plasma substitutes, European Health Committee, Council of Europe, Strasbourg, 1978.

PROCESSING CRITERIA FOR RECOVERY OF FFP FOR FRACTIONATION

J.K. Smith and D.R. Evans

Factor VIII is an expensive commodity when purchased on the international market. For reasons of economy, national self-respect and public health motives, many countries quite naturally wish to be self-sufficient from their own blood resources. Given a demand of about 30,000-60,000 IU per hemophiliac per year, or 2-4 IU per head of population per year; and given current yields of industrial-scale plasma processing between 120 and 250 IU per kg plasma, it is difficult to avoid the conclusion that factor VIII is now driving the national plasma and blood demand – not red cells, platelets or albumin. There must be a very high premium on improving the factor VIII coagulant yield from plasma, in order to save unnecessary collection of red cells which may be wasted.

In England, this realisation came at about the same time that our Medicines Inspectorate and the NBTS itself began taking a closer look at the way in which the NBTS separated and collected plasma for fractionation, the way in which cryoprecipitates were made and many aspects of production and quality control in large-scale processing at the national fractionation centres. Over the last four years, the production of cryoprecipitate in England and Wales has fallen off dramatically and the supply of plasma for fractionation has more than doubled. The average quality of that fresh frozen plasma has improved because it is now understood that the procurement of fresh frozen plasma is not a salvage operation; it must be carefully planned, costed and supported by the Transfusion Service.

One of the contributions the fractionators have helped to make is to look at the claims made for what makes plasma 'high quality' and to tell the Transfusion Centres which improvements might give the biggest return in terms of factor VIII yield. The Transfusion Centres know they will have returned to them factor VIII concentrate in proportion to the volume and quality of the plasma they send for fractionation and they are therefore keen to improve plasma quality at the lowest cost and disturbance to their existing practices.

What matters most economically, of course, is the yield of factor VIII delivered to the patient for every kilogram of FFP put into the system, but usually one has to draw inferences from comparisons made earlier in the process and even to see whether the yield is predictable from the factor VIII content of the plasma as it is frozen or as it goes into process. We will be talking mainly about the factor VIII content of plasma entering the process or the yield of concentrate after processing and freeze-drying (but before sampling for quality control). In a few cases it will be necessary to refer to data at the primary cyroprecipitate stage or before the finishing operations of sterile filtration dispensing and freeze-drying. Unless said otherwise, the process (1) used was the one established at Oxford seven years ago, or a minor variant of it (fig. 1). Different processing might promote the survival of a different selection of factor VIII molecules from the original plasma and no claims can be made for the universal application of our conclusions to different processes.

<u>100-300 kg FFP</u>

  │ Thaw 0-2°C
  ∨

<u>Cryoprecipitate</u>

  │ Extract in minimum vol. 0.02 M Tris, pH 7.0
  │ Absorb with Alhydrogel, centrifuge, filter
  ∨

<u>Adsorbed extract</u> (/4)

  │ Reduce pH to 6.6, temperature to 10°C
  ∨

<u>Cold supernatant</u>

  │ Adjust citrate, NaCl, pH (/5)
  │ Sterilise by 0.2 μ membrane filtration (/6)
  │ Dispense and freeze-dry
  ∨

<u>Final product</u> (/7)

Figure 1. Oxford process for factor VIII concentrate of intermediate specific activity.

Over the years we have seen a number of changes in the standard plasma delivered to Oxford and to Elstree. Initial data were obtained from 5 litre packs, containing about 28 donations of 180 ml, frozen vertically in an approximately 2" layer between two plates cooled to about -60°C, reaching a core temperature of about -30°C in less than two hours. Some of the data were checked later against single donations frozen in PVC bags over about 15 or 20 minutes, in vapour phase of liquid nitrogen and opened at the fractionation centre by dipping the frozen packs in liquid nitrogen. More recently, the dominant input to Elstree has been a new polyolefin pack designed primarily for mechanised opening at the fractionation plant. This wedge-shaped pack is frozen in a variety of ways at the Transfusion Centres and is opened straight out of the -30°C freezer by a custom built machine. Recently, Oxford has been looking intensively at Haemonetics and other plasmapheresis plasma, arriving like conventional plasma in larger PVC bags and more recently in a new bag designed for semi-automated tear-down. Some may have seen prototypes of a more highly developed machine at PFC in Edinburgh, designed to tear open specially adapted satellite packs.

ANTICOAGULANTS

Perhaps the most convincing improvement we have seen is in the factor VIII content of plasma taken into CPD rather than ACD anticoagulant and the survival of that difference throughout processing. In the 5 litre packs of plasma, sampled just before fractionation; in the extract of cryoprecipitate from about 100 kg of plasma; and in the freeze dried product, the difference was highly significant (table 1). We checked that this plasma difference was maintained througout a change-over from the 5 litre to PVC single donation packs. We attribute this difference to the inactivation of more factor VIII in the early stages of blood collection into a more acid anticoagulant medium (2). From time to time a Transfusion Centre has reverted to ACD in the hope of gaining some advantage in platelet recovery, and each time we have not needed to be told that they have made this change: the loss has been obvious from routine fractionation yields.

Table 1. Comparison of ACD and CPD anticoagulants: effect on plasma factor VIII and yield of intermediate concentrate

Samples for comparison	Factor VIII, IU/kg		
	ACD	CPD	Significance
Oxford 5 l packs 1978			
Plasma cores (n = 10)	710	810	Sign.
Cryo extract (n = 8)	325	367	Sign.
Final product (n = 8)	211	256	Sign.
Oxford SD packs 1979			
Plasma (n = 10)	710	805	Sign.

We have talked here about CPD, but in recent years most centres have moved to a CPD-A anticoagulant to get a longer shelf life for the red cells. Our date suggest that CPD-A is at least as good an anticoagulant for the preservation of factor VIII activity as plain CPD. There was a hint that CPD-A plasma performed slightly better but during the period in which we had both plasmas to fractionate, the difference did not reach 5% significance.

AGE

We originally set up analytical systems to examine plasma quality in response to a draft standard which would have put a four-hour limit on the interval between collecting blood and freezing it for coagulation factor production, a proposal which would have cut the amount of plasma delivered to English fractionation centres by more than 50 per cent, for an unquantified benefit. Table 2 shows, for Oxford plasma in 5 litre packs in either ACD or CPD anticoagulant, that although there is a small difference in plasma factor VIII between packs separated from blood centrifuged on the day of collection or on the morning after, the difference is not carried over into product yield. In this case, there is an apparent slight conflict of conclusions, since the Elstree laboratory finds a small but consistent difference of about 5 per cent in the yield from plasma from a different Transfusion Centre, separated on the same day or the day after collection, but the time bands are significantly different. We have not succeeded in getting sufficient plasma from the same Transfusion Centre for fractionation of several pools which were separated almost immediately after donation or early next day, but we do have some limited data on plasma factor VIII under these conditions (tabel 3). These are tantalising, suggesting that there may be an advantage to be gained from very rapid separation and freezing. That small difference may distinguish the two Regions concerned, one separating either very early on the day of donation and the other bringing back blood from a greater distance and separating usually about six to eight hours after donation on the same day.

The question was put to us, does the factor VIII concentrate from overnight plasma have the same immediate recovery and half-life in vivo as plasma separated within the same day? Our experience over 112 infusions (table 4) is that there is no significant difference in the patient's

Table 2. Factor VIII content of plasma in ACD and CPD anticoagulants, separated after 6-8 hours (FF) or after $\simeq$ 18 hours (ON); and the yield of concentrates derived from them.

| | Factor VIII recovery, IU/kg plasma | | | |
| | ACD | | CPD | |
	FF	ON	FF	ON
Cores of frozen packs (mean of 10 cores of 5 l packs)	720	700	840	770
Freeze-dried concentrate (mean of 8 batches)	214	208	255	257

Table 3. Factor VIII content of 5 litre plasma packs of different 'ages'

| Time (h) between blood collection and plasma freezing | Factor VIII (IU/kg) in plasma samples | | |
	(a) Before freezing pack	(b) After thawing pack to 20°C	(c) 'Core' sample of frozen pack
3-4 (special collection)	930	870	880
4-8 (routine FF)	840	820	790
16-18 (routine ON)	800	740	730

Mean of seven samples, ACD plasma, 2-stage VIII assay, plasma standard.

Table 4. Effect of whole blood (ACD) storage, before plasma separation, on patient 'response' to concentrates made from the plasma.

Oxford ACD plasma 1977, frozen over $\simeq$ 2h in 5l packs.
6 batches of concentrate made from each of two "ages" of plasma.
Factor VIII assays on patient plasma 1h after infusion.
(44 patients, 112 infusions).

Storage before separation	Mean patient respons = % rise x kg x IU infused^{-1}
6-8 hours	1.85
$\simeq$ 18 hours	2.13
	Not significant

immediate response but we cannot get hemophiliacs to co-operate as eagerly as they used to for the repeated visists necessary to get a half-disappearance.

PLASMA SEPARATION

We will look now at some claims for the importance of other variables. The Swiss Red Cross have reported (3) that fibrinopeptide A levels in plasma give a good reflection of efficient blood mixing during donation and that plasma pools with high FpA content do not fractionate as successfully as plasma with low FpA, from blood mixed very carefully during donation. This finding has not been confirmed in England or in Scotland by Prowse et al. (4), who believe that line-stripping may be more important than mixing. Our own feeling is that donation conditions in the field, and in the village hall, are very difficult to control and very variable from region to region and that if blood mixing were very influential in factor VIII recovery we would have seen this variable cutting across other correlations such as anticoagulant and age.

Again, some centres have specified double centrifugation of plasma, presumably in the hope of removing the last trace of cells from the plasma. We found no difference (table 5) in plasma factor VIII or cryo-precipitate factor VIII recovery between once- and twice-spun plasma, but of course a lot must depend on how efficiently one does the first separation. We do not like cells in plasma, but we would not recommend doubling spinning as an economic means of getting cleaner plasma or a higher factor VIII yield.

Table 5. Effect of doubling centrifugation of plasma on factor VIII.

Oxford ACD plasma 1975, single or double centrifugation, both 4000 x g angle rotor, 10 minutes.
Samples: 9 pools of 3 Group O + 3 Group A plasmas, and cryos made from these pools.

	Plasma IU/ml	Cryo IU/pack
Single centrifugation	0.96	96.3
Double centrifugation	0.99	91.8
	Not significant	Not significant

PACK SIZE, FREEZING RATE

Within certain limits, we think that many efficient ways of freezing plasma are adequate for factor VIII recovery. A lot of time and money has been spent promoting very rapid freezing, but we have to look at what 'slow' freezing method the rapid freezing method is being compared with. If one throws 20 kilograms of randomly packed, ovoid plasma bags into the top of an inefficient domestic freezer, or even a walk-in freezer with a heavy warm load, it may take 10-20 hours for the centre of the pack to reach -25°C and one will see a loss of factor VIII, compared with a 10 mm layer of plasma held between plates cooled to -80°C. However, when we compared reasonably practical ways of freezing in less than 2 hours, so that the day's plasma supply was processed rapidly enough, we did not see a significant difference in plasma factor VIII or recovery in concentrate (table 6).

Table 6. Effect of pack type and rate of freezing on plasma factor VIII.

   (a) Oxford CPD plasma, 1979; separated after 6-8 h or ≃ 18 h,
       pooled and frozen in 5 l packs over ≃ 2 h.
   (b) Oxford CPD plasma, 1979; separated after 6-8 h or ≃ 18 h,
       frozen single in vapour phase over liquid N_2, ≃ 15 min.
   Samples: (a) Cores of 5 l packs.
              (b) Pool of cores from 2 Group O + 2 Group A plasmas.

Freezing	Plasma IU/ml	
	6-8 hours	18 hours
5 l packs over ≃ 2 h	0.84 ± 0.13	0.77 ± 0.08 (n=10)
SD packs over ≃ 15 min.	0.86 ± 0.10	0.77 ± 0.15 (n=10)
	Not significant	Not significant

We have seen no significant improvement in the factor VIII supply from freezing very thin layers or thick layers, say 10-15 mm compared with about 50 mm, provided freezing to -30° in the core was achieved within a few hours. We have seen 10-20% losses of plasma factor VIII in plasma attributable to placing a load of plasma in an overworked freezer with a lot of other warm material and left to freeze overnight, or taken out of an efficient freezer when the outer skin had just frozen and placed in a "conserving" freezer when it might even re-melt for a time.

TEMPERATURE OF STORAGE

For strategic reasons, fractionators often wish to store FFP for consider-able periods before fractionation. Within recent memory in England, some of the reasons have been
1. Pooling of plasma by single region or by type, for example anticoagulant or age, to encourage improvements in plasma quality.
2. Quarantine against later reports of hepatitis in donors.
3. Stockpiling during plant renewal or building up capacity.
The Oxford laboratory has always adopted a standard temperature lower than -30°C for storage of FFP, -40°C when possible, and all freezers are set to alarm when the outer layer of stored plasma would reach that temperature of -30°C. We have fractionated several pools of plasma initially quarantined after some query about safety or identity, and stored for more than one year below -30°C before fractionation. The overall yield of factor VIII concentrate has been within the usual range for plasma stored for only a few weeks. We have no data on starting plasma factor VIII, so this might be an example of excellent cryoprecipitation and survival during processing, like the twice-frozen plasma to be discussed later. The PFC in Edinburgh has evidence that the longer plasma is stored in the frozen state, the more fibrinogen is precipitated

in the cryoprecipitate. This effect has not been confirmed in England, possibly because of differences in plasma storage patterns, cryoprecipitate production, extraction and purification techniques. The stability of factor VIII in plasma, and especially its ultimate recovery in concentrate, are obviously subject of many recognised and unrecognised variables, and no-one really wants to store hundreds of kilograms of plasma deliberately at temperatures between -20°C and -25°C to prove the point, but it does seem to use that at -30°C time stands still for the factor VIII recoverable by our kind of process.

This represents a temperature below -25°C which is loosely said to be one of the 'eutectic' points of freezing plasma, but those who are versed in the necromancy of freeze-drying will know that there are other inflections in the conductivity versus temperature curve between -20°C and -40°C, and possibly beyond, so any recourse to theory is probably fruitless.

We have already shown one example relating to plasma age, that differences in plasma are not always reflected in the yield of concentrate. Here is another extreme example. For operational reasons, one Transfusion Centre was freezing single donations of plasma on the day of donation and thawing them the next day for pooling into 5 litre packs and refreezing. This process, not unexpectedly, approximately halved the original factor VIII content of the plasma (table 7). However, the proportion of factor VIII that did survive was extremely well recovered by cryoprecipitation and through the rest of the fractionation process, so that the final yield was indistinguishable from once-frozen plasma from the same region over the same period — not the best quality, but still very well worth processing. One suspects that the main explanation was not the stability of the surviving factor VIII but changes in factor VIII, fibrinogen and fibronectin proteins promoting the very efficient cryoprecipitation of factor VIII.

Table 7. Effect of thawing and re-freezing CPD plasma on plasma factor VIII and yield from concentrate

(a) Wessex plasma separated within ≃ 8 h of donation, frozen in single satellite packs; then thawed, pooled into 5 l packs and re-frozen.
(b) Wessex plasma separated after ≃ 18 h and pooled directly into 5 l packs, frozen over ≃ 2 h.
Samples: (i) 'Cores' of SD or 5 l packs.
         (ii) Stages to intermediate purity (concentrate, 8 CRV).

Stage	Stage yield IU/kg		Difference
	Once-frozen	Twice-frozen	
Plasma cores (plasma standard)	593 ± 99	301 ± 116	Sign.
Cryo extract (conc. standard)	330 ± 35	291 ± 35	Not sign.
Dried product	194 ± 19	192 ± 19	Not sign.

We would like to confirm that excellent plasma for fractionation of factor VIII can be recovered by machine plasmapheresis techniques. About half of Oxford's plasma input, approximately 5000 kg per year, is now in the form of Haemonetics or other plasmapheresis plasma, collected by various techniques and in various anticoagulants. We have summarised 16 months' data from Oxford (table 8).

1. Haemonetics cryoprecipitate tends to be a little heavier than that from conventional plasma recovered by spinning whole blood in bags. We have to work a little harder to extract this factor VIII but it is worthwhile.

Table 8. Process yields etc. for conventional and Haemonetics plasma, PFL, March 1983–June 1984.

Separation method	Anti- coagulant	Region	n	g cryoppt per kg plasma	Factor VIII plasma	IU/kg
					Extract	Pre-finish
Manual < 18 h	CPDA	F	13	9.1 ± 0.5	391 ± 31	290 ± 25
Haemonetics	CPD	C	16	10.8 ± 1.1	461 ± 50	319 ± 33

2. Yields of factor VIII in cryoprecipitate and after processing are significantly higher than from conventional plasma, probably because of earlier freezing.

Although it is possible that we could take still greater advantage of the high factor VIII in Haemonetics pools at the cryoprecipitate stage by more selective processing of this grade of plasma rather than just applying the usual standard process, data so far suggest that the percentage stage losses are very similar for both Haemonetics and conventional plasma.

Finally, we must not forget that there are other valuable proteins besides factor VIII to be recovered from plasma, and our considerations of 'quality' should not ignore them. One good example from the Haemonetics program can be given, showing that the method of collecting plasma may influence the quality of factor IX recovered. We have found that the non-activated partial thromboplastin times (NAPTT) of batches prepared from Haemonetics pools are significantly shorter than those from conventional pools made at about the same time (table 9).

Table 9. Factor IX (II, X) from conventional and Haemonetics plasma.

	NAPTT 1/10 (sec)	Factor IX IU/kg
Conventional plasma n = 21	230 ± 27	388 ± 56
Haemonetics plasma n = 7	194 ± 26	443 ± 46

It is possible that this difference reflects a higher concentration of platelets, of soluble platelet products or even of soluble red cell products in machine collected plasma, and we are looking forward to the imminent advent of filter apheresis plasma, hopefully completely free of all cellular contamination.

REFERENCES

1. Smith JK, Evans DR, Stone V, Snape TJ. A factor VIII concentrate of intermediate purity and higher potency. Transfusion 1979;19:299-306.
2. Vermeer C, Soute BAM, Ates G, Brummelhuis HGJ. Contributions to the optimal use of human blood. VII. Increase of the yield of factor VIII in four-donor cryoprecipitate by an improved processing of blood and plasma. Vox Sang 1976;30:1-22.
3. Pflugshaupt R, Kurt G. FpA content — a criterion of quality for plasma as factor VIII source. Vox Sang 1983;45:224-32.
4. Prowse CV, Bessos H, Farrugia A, Smith A, Gabra J. Donation procedure, fibrinopeptide A and factor VIII. Vox Sang 1984;46:55-7.

DONATION PROCEDURE: COLLECTION LESION, FIBRINOPEPTIDE A, AND FACTOR VIII

C.V. Prowse

Following the work of Pflugshaupt (1) a number of groups, including ourselves have re-investigated the effects of donation procedures on the quality of plasma destined for preparation of factor VIII concentrates. The Swiss group argued that thrombin formation in donated blood might have two adverse effects on the quality of plasma; firstly degradation of factor VIII yielding a more labile product, and secondly generation of fibrin resulting in a less soluble product, if this protein forms part of the final factor VIII concentrate. Using fibrinopeptide A (FpA) levels as a measure of the presence of thrombin, they confirmed that plasma containing more than 50 ng/ml FpA resulted in a poorly soluble and labile product when the factor concentrate was made by their technique. It was also shown that an improved donation procedure could reduce plasma FpA levels.

FpA is released from fibrinogen during the formation of fibrin by thrombin. It is determined by radioimmunoassay which reveals basal levels of < 2 ng/ml upon careful collection in a heparin-based anticoagulant to inhibit thrombin. Citrate based anticoagulants will not prevent this action of thrombin, although preventing thrombin generation. Plasma antithrombins will however inhibit formed thrombin within a few minutes. Serum levels of FpA are about 20,000 ng/ml, thus a plasma level of 50 ng/ml corresponds to about 0.2% conversion of fibrinogen to fibrin or 5 mg/l fibrin. This is in itself insoluble but may also form poorly soluble complexes in association with native fibrinogen. The actions of low levels of thrombin on plasma factor VIII are less easy to determine due to the wide range of factor VIII in the normal population and the inaccuracy of the currently available assays.

In our studies we chose to perform model experiments, on relatively small numbers of donations to look at specific aspects of the donation procedure, and determined factor VIII and FpA levels as a measure of plasma quality. FpA was assayed by Nossel's method using the original dialysis technique to separate FpA from cross-reacting fibrinogen (2), and IMCO reagents. In preliminary experiments we showed that while plasma from donated blood contains higher amounts of FpA than the basal amounts described above, as has been shown by others (1,3), addition of the usual heparin-aprotinin cocktail had no benefit (fig. 1). This was true even for plasma containing elevated levels of FpA. In all subsequent work we have therefore assessed normal CPD-A plasma as such. This is, after all, the material used in preparing factor VIII concentrates. We also found that storage of blood or plasma overnight resulted in little if any increase in FpA levels (fig. 2). Similar results have been reported from Dr. Akerblom's group (3,4) who have extended their observation to plasma stored in plastic packs at 4°C for longer periods. FpA levels remained stable up to 14 days but rose thereafter, possibly due to cold-activation of factors VII and XII, an effect that was more pronounced in ACD-Terumo units than CPD-Fenwal units (4). This effect is obviously of minor interest to factor VIII producers who usually only fractionate plasma frozen within a day of donation.

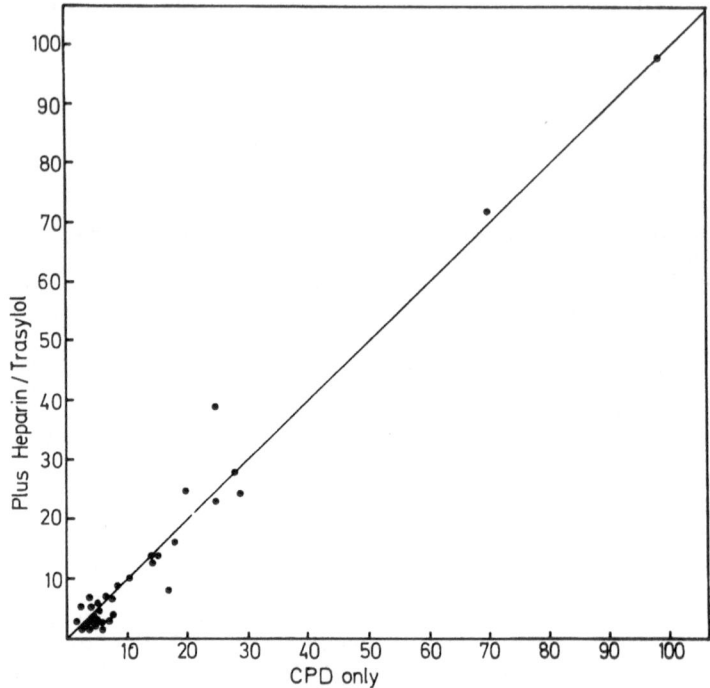

Figure 1. Effect of inhibitors on donor plasma FpA (ng/ml).
FpA (ng/ml) levels in CPD plasma from normal donations with or without
additon of 100 μ/ml each of heparin and aprotinin prior to freezing for
later assay (n=33, r=0.998, p < 0.001).

Our initial interest was whether our standard donation procedure,
involving gentle manual mixing at approximately minute intervals with
blood entering the inverted pack through the anticoagulant, produced
plasma of a poorer quality than that which might be obtained by a more
rigorous procedure, corresponding to the effect of an automated donation mixer. As reported recently (5) we carried out two separate studies
in different centres and found no benefit, in terms of FpA or factor
VIII, of additional mixing. Average FpA levels were actually lower in
blood that was not mixed until the end of donation (fig. 3), in apparent
contrast to the results obtained in Switzerland (1). In passing it is
worth mentioning that Professor Walter states, in a recent review of the
development of plastic blood bags, 'it became possible to collect blood
by gravity into an empty blood bag and refrigerate it for 6-8 h without
clotting'. In similar vein, Kasper (7) found it necessary to store unmixed
blood totally undisturbed for 4 h at 20°C to demonstrate a significant
drop in cryoprecipitate factor VIII. Our first study also led to two
secondary conclusions. A trend towards increased FpA levels with longer
donation times was noted, which became significant for donations taking
longer than 10 minutes. This may be inherent in the longer donation
times but is more likely to be due to the quality of the vein and vene-
puncture resulting in both a raised FpA level and the slow flow of blood.
In addition the mean FpA level obtained in the two studies differed
significantly (fig. 3). This was ascribed to differences in the care paid

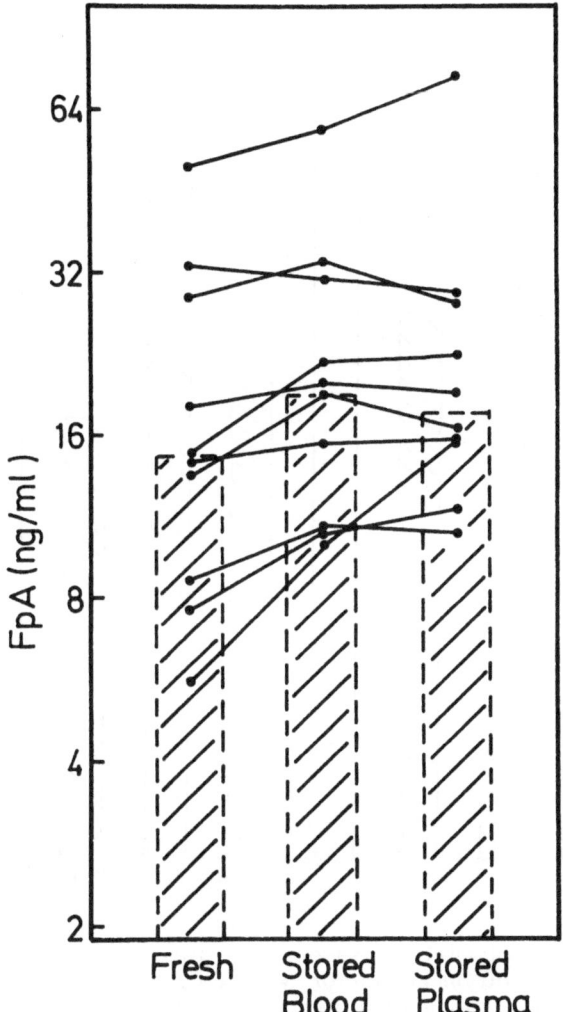

Figure 2. Effect of storage on blood and plasma FpA.
FpA levels (ng/ml) in aliquots from 10 standard donations assayed on
plasma frozen immediately and after 20 h storage at 20°C as blood or
plasma. Shaded columns show median values, which did not differ
significantly (Wilcoxon test).

in promptly stripping donation lines (5), but it must be admitted that
other less obvious differences existed between the two studies such as
the type of pack used (Tuta and Fenwal) and the delay between donation
and plasma separation.
Carlebjork has reported slightly higher levels of FpA in stripped donor
lines than in the blood bag itself (3). While both the above studies were
specially performed it must be emphasized that assay of our routine frozen
plasma product reveals similar levels of FpA (fig. 4) and factor VIII.

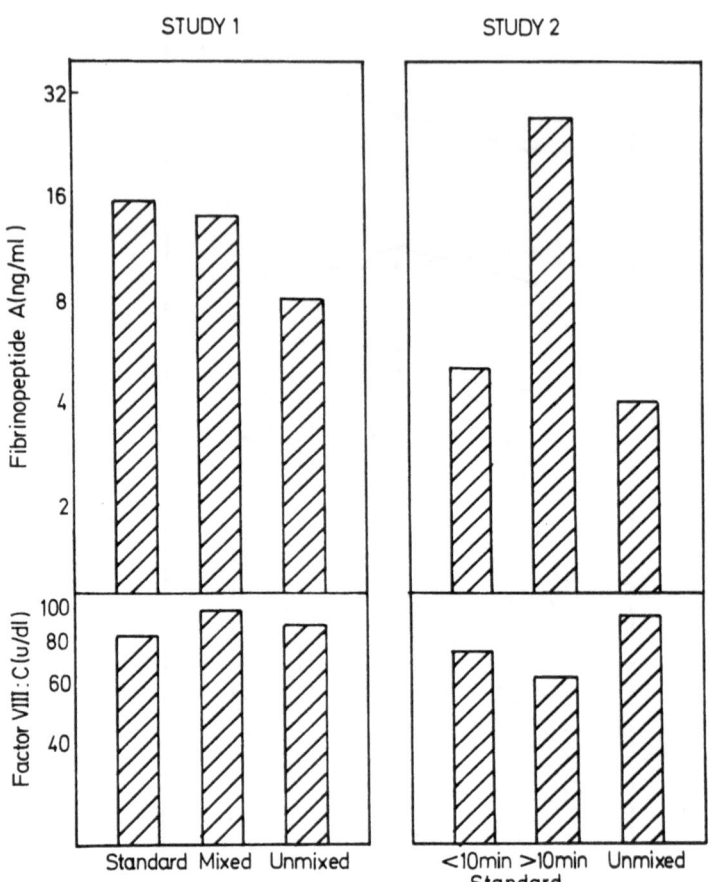

Figure 3. Effect of mixing and donation time on plasma FpA.
Median FpA (ng/ml) and mean factor VIII (IU/ml) for 10 donations in
each group. During donations in study 1 blood was manually mixed each
minute during collection in an inverted pack (standard), continously
manually mixed (mixed) or not mixed until the end of donation, the
pack being placed upright (unmixed). Tuta CPD-A packs were used.
Mean donation time was 5.3 minutes for 450 ml blood. In study 2 the
same standard and unmixed procedures were used, but 10 donations
were also collected by the standard procedure but with donation times
in excess of 10 minutes. This resulted in a significant increase in FpA
($p < 0.01$). Fenwal CPD-A packs were used.

In a follow up study, carried out in co-operation with Dr. Robinson
in Leeds, we have assessed FpA levels and platelet contamination in
plasma obtained by different apheresis procedures. Despite the fact that
such collections involve metered addition of anticoagulant with the blood
as soon as it leaves the vein, FpA levels did not differ appreciably from
those obtained in standard donations. This applied whether platelet rich
– or platelet poor – plasma procedures were used (fig. 4). Somewhat

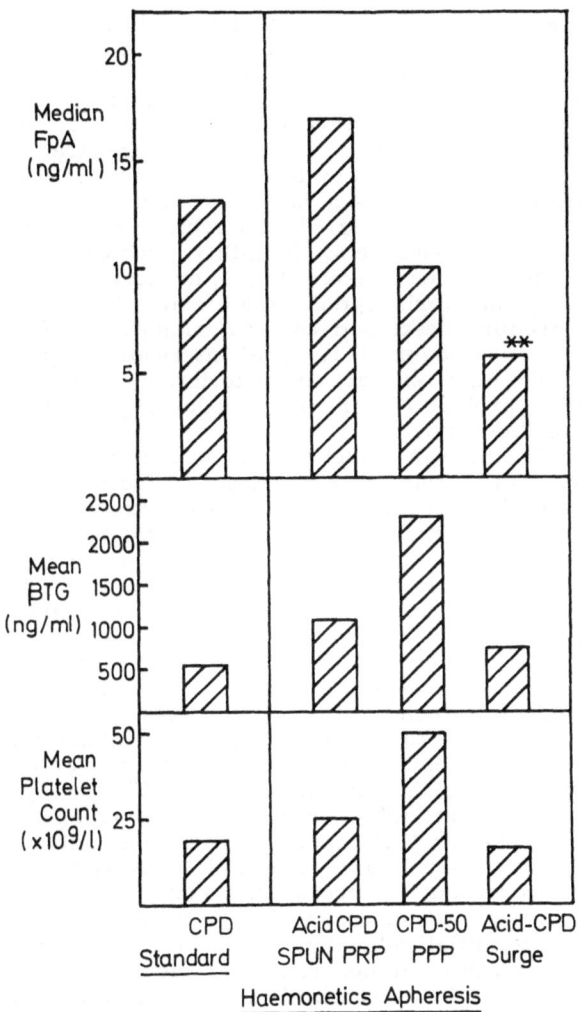

Figure 4. Quality of plasma obtained by apheresis.
FpA, beta-thromboglobulin and platelet count in plasma from standard CPD-A donations (n > 200) and in plasma obtained by Haemonetics apheresis using platelet poor (PPP), platelet rich (PRP, subsequently re-centrifuged) and surge techniques with the indicated anticoagulants. n ≥ 10 in each group. **: FpA levels were significantly lower in surge plasma than in apheresis plasma obtained by the other two apheresis protocols (p < 0.02).

lower FpA levels were noted in plasma collected by the 'surge' technique which also contained fewer platelets. Our conclusions from these experiments are that, provided donations are taken in under 10 minutes and mixed a few times during donation by manual or automated methods, FpA levels do not reach levels that have been associated with problems in preparing factor VIII concentrates, although occasional individual donations show elevated levels. On this basis the assay of FpA as a criterion for plasma quality would appear to be more applicable in assessing novel procedures rather than for routine use.

Due to the problems mentioned above, the effect of donation procedure on plasma factor VIII is more difficult to assess. Useful data may be obtained by assessing factor VIII products prepared from selected plasma pools. Recent work from Finland (8), using a novel method of factor VIII purification, suggests a labile product was only found when plasma FpA levels exceeded 100 ng/ml. To achieve this it was necessary to add thrombin to the plasma pool. Solubility problems were apparently not encountered and it seems likely that purification procedures that remove the majority of fibrin(ogen) from factor VIII may avoid such difficulties. The product described by Pflugshaupt contains a relatively high proportion of fibrinogen (1). The intermediate purity products produced in the UK have similar characteristics, but we very rarely encounter solubility problems with this product, prepared from plasma of the quality described above.

We have also used the FpA model system to approach another problem area in factor VIII procurement — the loss of factor VIII between the time of donation and the freezing of plasma. Collection of blood in normal citrate anticoagulants results in an initial loss of up to 10% of factor VIII due to acid insults as the first portion of blood enters the anticoagulant (9), followed by a further loss of up to 50% of activity over the next 20 hours as a result of calcium chelation (10,11). Both problems may be reduced by collection in heparin anticoagulant (11,12), and further improvements may be achieved by addition of extra calcium (13). While this approach has been successfully applied in Groningen to the production of freeze-dried cryoprecipitate on a relatively small scale (12), there are problems in the large scale processing of heparinised plasma (14,15). This is possibly due to heparin-induced precipitation of fibronectin and might be avoided by use of heparin derivatives. The study of Mikaelsson (13) suggested to us that collection in reduced strength citrate might also provide greater factor VIII stability. Red cells collected in reduced strength citrate solution are known to exhibit improved quality (16,17).

A preliminary experiment confirmed that factor VIII stability in blood was improved, compared to standard CPD anticoagulant, by addition of some calcium, or by initial collection in heparin (table 1). Addition of calcium to heparin plasma further improved factor VIII stability, while addition of citrate was only detrimental at concentrations above 10 mM.

Table 1. Effect of additives on plasma factor VIII:C stability.

Plasma type	Addition	% initial factor VIII:C	
		at 6 h	at 20 h
CPD plasma	none	74 ± 22	61 ± 11
	10 mM $CaCl_2$ + 2 u/ml Heparin	-	81 ± 14
	20 mM $CaCl_2$ + 2 u/ml Heparin	-	83 ± 13
Heparin plasma	none	100 ± 28	78 ± 17
	10 mM citrate	-	78 ± 8
	20 mM citrate	-	55 ± 1
	10 mM $CaCl_2$	-	96 ± 13

All values are final concentrations. Mean ± SD for six experiments.

Table 2. Plasma quality following collection in CPD dilutions.

Final plasma citrate (mM)	VIII:C at 22 h (IU/dl)	FpA (ng/ml) (median)	Ionised Ca^{2+} (uM)	BTG (ng/ml)	pH
20 (neat CPD)	68 ± 17	40	25	1445	7.6
16	71 ± 13	30	36	1243	7.7
12	80 ± 16	28	61	1313	7.7
10	76 ± 20	25	77	1275	7.7
8	86 ± 17	17	96	975	7.7
4	Clot at 30 m	13,350	276	3450	7.8
Heparin	92 ± 22	23	955	1647	7.9

7 ml blood was collected in 1 ml of different dilutions of CPD in phosphate dextrose. Mean of six experiments (± SD): Blood was left at 20°C for 22 h prior to VIII:C assay.

Standard CPD anticoagulant yields plasma containing about 20 mM citrate, for donors with a 45% hematocrit. On this basis we collected blood from six volunteers and aliquoted this into various dilutions of CPD in 16 mM disodium phosphate, 129 mM dextrose. Table 2 shows that, compared to standard CPD, no difference in FpA level was found until plasma citrate levels fell below 8 mM, when gross clotting occurred. Between 8 and 12 mM citrate a significant increase in factor VIII stability was noted. These citrate levels correspond to plasma ionised calcium levels of 60 to 100 µM and did not result in increased platelet release, as determined by radioimmunoassay of beta-thromboglobulin. It remains to be seen if half strength CPD is an adequate anticoagulant for general use and is compatible with bulk plasma fractionation.

ACKNOWLEDGEMENTS

I would like to thank my collaborators in these studies, in particular H. Bessos, J. Dawes, A. Farrugia, J. Gabra and A. Robinson. Any conclusions are, however, my own.

REFERENCES

1. Pfugshaupt R, Kurt G. FpA content — a criterion of quality for plasma factor VIII source. Vox Sang 1983;45:224-32.
2. Nossel HL, Yudelmann I, Canfield RE, et al. Measurement of fibrinopeptide A in human blood. J Clin Invest 1974;54:43-53.
3. Carlebjork G, Blomback M, Akerblom O. Improvement of plasma quality as raw material for factor VIII concentrates: storage of whole blood and plasma and interindividual plasma levels of fibrinopeptide A. Vox Sang 1983;45:233-42.
4. Blomback M, Chmielewska J, Netre C, Akerblom O. Activation of blood coagulation, fibrinolytic and kallikrein systems during storage of plasma. Vox Sang 1984;47:335-42.

5. Prowse CV, Bessos H, Farrugia A, Smith A, Gabra J. Donation procedure, fibrinopeptide A and factor VIII. Vox Sang 1984;46:55-7.
6. Walter CW. Invention and development of the blood bag. Vox Sang 1984;47:318-24.
7. Kasper CK, Myhre BA, McDonald JD, Nakasako Y, Feinstein DI. Determinants of factor VIII recovery in cryoprecipitate. Transfusion 1975;15:312-22.
8. Torma E, Myllyla G. Parameters affecting the fractionation of factor VIII:C activity in production of very high purity AHF concentrate. Scan J Haematol 1984;33(Suppl 40):123-6.
9. Vermeer C, Soute BAM, Ates G, Hellings JA, Brummelhuis HGJ. Contributions to the optimal use of human blood: VIII: Stability of blood coagulation factor VIII during collection and storage of whole blood and plasma. Vox Sang;31(Suppl 1):55-67.
10. Weiss HJ. A study of the cation and pH-dependant stability of factors V and VIII in plasma. Thromb Diath Haemorrh 1965;14:32-51.
11. Rock GA, Cruickshank WH, Tackaberry ES, Palmer DS. Improved yields of factor VIII from heparinised plasma. Vox Sang 1979;36:294-300.
12. Smit Sibinga CTh, Das PC. Heparin and factor VIII. Scand J Haematol 1984;33(Suppl 40):111-26.
13. Mikaelsson ME, Forsman N, Oswaldsson UM. Human Factor VIII: a calcium-linked protein complex. Blood 1983;62:1006-15.
14. Smith JK qu in Penny AF. Anticoagulation in cell separation procedures. Apheresis Bulletin 1983;1:164-71.
15. Margolis J, Gallovich CM, Rhoades P. A process for preparation of 'high purity' factor VIII by controlled pore glass treatment. Vox Sang 1984;46:341-8.
16. Loutit JF. Factors influencing the preservation of stored red cells. J Pathol 1945;57:325-35.
17. Mishler JM, Darley JH, Haworth C, Mollison PL. Viability of red cells stored in diminished concentration of citrate. Br J Haematol 1979;43:63-7.

DISCUSSION

Moderators: S. Seidl en J. Over

D.H. Naylor (Toronto):

I would just like to make a comment. In our country, we have had a plasmapheresis program for the last three or four years. Our difficulties have not been in convincing donors to contribute on a voluntary basis, however the difficulty has been in trying to convince funding authorities to supply the money to increase our collections.

S. Seidl (Frankfurt am Main):

There is a special system in Canada. For those who are not familiar with it, all blood is collected by the Canadian Red Cross, of course non-remunerated, and is distributed to the hospitals free of charge. The money for all processing costs comes in from the Government. I am explaining this to you, because in some countries, other systems do exist. In Germany, we do likewise. We collect blood non-remunerated, but we add our processing fees before distributing the blood to the hospitals. Would someone like to say something on this?

H.H. Gunson (Manchester):

I think it is a difficulty to get the capital investment to produce the plasma, because you have a lag phase between putting that investment in and getting the benefits of the products from your own plasma. National Health authorities are reluctant to purchase commercial products during the time in which you have to build up the plasma supply. It is a difficulty; if you can get over it, the benefits come back later on.

F. Peetoom (Portland):

In the United States, some companies are actually preparing for a decline in the demand for plasma fractionation from the paid plasma donors. This is why, for instance, Hyland Laboratories, a subsidiary of Baxter Travenol, has made an agreement with the National American Red Cross to have the majority of the volunteer donor plasma fractionated at the company under contract. This has allowed them to expand or upgrade their facilities, because they are guaranteed under this agreement that whatever growth in the plasma production in the volunteer Red Cross sector will be fractionated on their premises. And so they are dealing with the same problem. But certain provisions have been made to make these improvements through capital investment possible because of a guaranteed supply. I think that other countries that see also recombinant

DNA proteins on the horizon, have a new disincentive to make lots of money available for upgrading of this processing capability.

C.Th. Smit Sibinga (Groningen):

Dr. Peetoom, your presentation was most exciting. Some may now have the idea that there is no longer any future in blood banking, but I think we will survive.

I do have some questions with regard to your manificent scheme for the future. First of all the chemical substitutes: There have been many rumors over the past couple of years about chemicals. It has even been named artificial blood. However, it is evident from your scheme that it is only a minute part. Could you give us some information on what you think, what kind of chemicals and what functions of the blood they will represent or will replace in the near future? We know about the fluoro-carbons, we know about some of the hemoglobins to be made out of red cells and then altered and changed chemically, but maybe you have some other things to tell us?

The second point is: When we see the basic blood supply decreasing gradually from time level two on down to time level four, what do you think will be the role for Blood Banks in the future? This definitely leads to the disappearance of Blood Centres. It might lead to an increase in size of some of the Blood Banks which eventually will survive. But these will have to change their techniques, their processing attitudes, etc. to deal with these new techniques in the future. Do you see the Blood Banking community getting involved in the production of, for instance, recombinant DNA, or the cell culture techniques, or maybe the refining of commercially prepared raw materials, cells, etc.? Do you see any specific future in new storage techniques, as these products might have different circumstances for survival and eventually for issuing to the clinic?

F. Peetoom:

The chemical segment of the box — I appreciate you reminding me that I did not touch on that. I feel that anything chemical that tends to be removed in its basic structure from our own biological structure, causes problems, or requires a clinical compromise. We know that fluosol, for instance, is seen by our defense cells as a foreign substance. All these cells that phagocytize throw themselves on these particles to the point where our defense system, which can be demonstrated as unable to react against virus or bacterial organisms, is at least temporarily paralyzed. There is preoccupation of our immune system with foreign materials — fluosol is a foreign material, so would other chemical substitutes be. I am in favour of the real biological substance of compatible nature. We know now that fluosol is not going to be promoted any longer as a substitute for red cells in acute or chronic anemias. Fluosol, to replace red cells for general transfusion has been given up, because of side effects. Nevertheless, there are two new applications for fluosol in the United States: One is to facilitate angioplasty, which is the widening of narrowed coronary arteries; by putting little balloons into those vessels and inflating them up to expand the vessel wall to increase the lumen. By leading a thin tubing through those balloons carrying oxygenated fluosol, one can oxygenate the heart muscle distally from those little balloons. This permits angioplasty to be performed during many more minutes than just the intermittent few minutes, as could be done before. So, this procedure is much more effective with fluosol.

Another application with fluosol is in the oxygenation of blood vessel poor tumors. The effect of chemotherapy and irradiation increases with the metabolic activity of the tumor cells which is supported by improved oxygen supply, provided by hyper-oxygenated fluosol. So, there will now be specific clinical applications for these chemical substitutes, but those will not haunt us in our general transfusion practices. The future of a Blood Centre depends on the imagination of its leadership, and on the community support that it has in performing its functions. Economics, obviously, are a major issue in the survival of Blood Centres and Blood Banks; we will have to be very imaginative to assume new roles. If we have not put some money away to take care of this, our capital reserves; if we do not have the talents, we will fall by the wayside. I believe there will be more regionalisation, there will be more regional services. Cost effectiveness and efficiency will be major factors. It is an uncertain future, and the capabilities of the people running the Blood Centres will be crucial.

There are many opportunities, but it is the people who have to initiate them and they have to have a lot of support, or develop new working structures. In the Netherlands, you have all the elements to succeed together. However, frequently, human relationships make these opinions fail or succeed.

S. Seidl:

One further question regarding what has already been said. When it comes to genetic engineering, it has been calculated that the space you need to provide the whole world with Factor VIII could be easily contained in this room. The question is: Is there a place in the Blood Bank for genetic engineering?

Secondly, you have also been talking about cultivating cells, instead of using fluosol for carrying oxygen. Is red cell cultivation feasible in 30 to 40 years?

F. Peetoom:

It is currently possible to drive stem cells to the nucleated stage of red cell differentiation. The crucial trick which is necessary to develop this into an industrial-scale process requires the disclosure of the biochemical processes involved in cloning, so that these cells can be cloned. It is impossible to produce enough red cells for transfusion by fifty divisions which most cells go through. That is a little bottle of blood.

The biochemical understanding of cloning will allow us to generate large amounts of cells. Obviously, this is not on level two, this comes at level three of the chart I showed. I have indicated that this will be considerably further removed than taking care of plasma protein needs.

J.A. Loos (Amsterdam):

Dr. Peetoom, you showed the effort a Blood Centre has to put into the several aspects of the Blood Bank in the near future. You mentioned that there will be quite a big increase of effort in the processing of the blood. My question is: Is this related to economics, or is this related to labour, for I think that 'robotising' the total process in the Blood Bank will reduce human effort in preparing components.

F. Peetoom:

I may have omitted mentioning the total resource allocation on future time level four. I indicated that the laboratory, or technical services in blood processing would gain in absolute and relative size. So, .whatever the dollar allocation is today, ignoring inflation and so forth, there would still be growth. Indeed, this is not due to the increased volume of whole blood being processed into cryoprecipitate, platelets, etcetera. It is due to the central role that the laboratory can play in the future in providing a multitude of services to a regional system. I feel that with the technologies, the skills and the proficiency of the staffs, there are many services that can be provided cheaper by regional centres to regional hospitals. This trend will not decline, but will rather increase.

There will, also, be additional testing need and there will be more complex compatibility issues. Not so much with red cells, because there will be less immunisation from a universal donor red cell type produced in vitro. There will be more compatibility testing for bone marrow and certain other cells. It is a replacement activity in the laboratory which will still lead to activity growth rather than decline in Blood Centres that take a pro-active attitude.

J.P.H.B. Sybesma (Dordrecht):

Dr. Gunson, is DDAVP already used in the U.K. during plasmapheresis procedures of donors?

H.H. Gunson:

No, it is not. I am putting it forward really just as a possibility. It has been used largely on an experimental basis in Sweden. But I am not aware of widespread use of it. If you are going to give this substance repeatedly, one has to be very careful, that the side effects are not a contra-indication in the long term.

F. Peetoom:

Dr. Prowse, as an immunologist I am concerned about the negative effects of immuno-modulation from blood transfusion through the presence of lymphocytes with many antigens that go to work in the recipient. I wonder if you have any opinion about the presence of lymphocyte surface antigens in cryoprecipitate products, or non-purified cryoprecipitate products, their contribution to immuno-suppression in hemophiliac recipients, and whether this in itself might be a reason to demand more purified products rather than less purified products.

C.V. Prowse (Edingburgh):

I cannot answer that specifically. We have been doing some in vitro work with suppression of lymphocyte transformation by Factor VIII products.

This follows published work from Glasgow (1). It is known that Factor VIII products can suppress in vitro lymphocyte function. We can get rid of that activity just by dialysing the FVIII concentrate, so it is unlikely that it is the FVIII itself that is an immuno-suppressive component.

F. Peetoom:

What is your activity loss when you dialyse Factor VIII concentrate?

C.V. Prowse:

Depends how you do it. It can be up to 30%, but is more usually around 10%.

A.S. Harris (Malmø):

In Sweden, as part of a national program to make the country self-sufficient in source plasma for Factor VIII preparations, the possibility was investigated of improving the yield and quality by means of DDAVP administration to blood donors. The efficacy of this procedure has been reported in many publications. On the safety side, I just want to add that in over 400 donors who have been followed over a long period of time, we have looked into the transient side effects such as occasional flushing that one sees with effect of DDAVP intranasally. Moreover, in addition approximately 40 donors were closely monitored during twice monthly plasma donations after DDAVP stimulation for 9 months. Here we have also looked into its effect on clinical laboratory parameters such as blood status, plasma proteins, liver enzymes as well as the effects on other blood coagulation factors. After long term repeated intermittent use of DDAVP intranasally, we have documentary evidence that there are no significant effects of the drug on these parameters, with the exception of increased yields and purity of Factor VIII (2).

J. Over (Amsterdam):

Dr. Prowse, I was not quite sure about the significance of the decrease of the FVIII related antigen in the cryo after slow freezing. I was amazed to see this.

C.V. Prowse:

This relates specifically to cryoprecipitate made by the thaw syphon process. It seems to be particularly susceptible to flaking off the cryo-precipitate which finds its way into the supernatant.

1. Froebel KS, Madhok R, Forbes CD, Lennie SE, Lowe GDO, Sturrock RD. Immunological abnormalities in haemophilia — are they caused by American factor VIII concentrate?. Brit Med J 1983;287:1091-3.
2. Jonsson S, Harris AS, Nilsson IM. A long term study on the efficacy and safety of administration of DDAVP in repeated plasma donation. Xth Congress of the International Society on Thrombosis and Haemostasis San Diego, 1985.

J. Over:

So, the composition of the cryo was different, compared to fast-frozen plasma? Is it a matter of flocculation of proteins?

C.V. Prowse:

Are we comparing fast and slow?

J. Over:

Yes.

C.V. Prowse:

In the actual mass of proteins, there is not that much difference. It is about half fibrinogen, a third fibronectin and the rest is general plasma protein. But this is only because FVIII is a very small-mass protein, in terms of the weight in a litre of plasma.

F. Peetoom:

I would like to hear somebody's opinion as to what might be behind these controversial results. Why is FVIII obviously a stable component by many criteria and not so in some people's hands.

J.K. Smith (Oxford):

What is the controversy about? About the stability under different conditions?

F. Peetoom:

Unless I have missed the point, there seems to be definite consensus that FVIII can hardly be damaged by any of the variables that it can go through in different environments, collection agencies, processing and so forth. At the same time, there is a lot of variety of opinion as to how to avoid damage to FVIII, some people even say it does not matter much what you do. What seems to be the major cause for this variety of opinions at the present time: is FVIII stable or is it not stable?

J.K. Smith:

No fractionator would like to give the impression that one can do anything one likes with fresh frozen plasma and still have a good result. I think everyone likes to see some limits put on the degree of injury that you subject plasma to. What we have been trying to do is shore up the limits of the abuse to which you can put FFP and expect to get good FVIII from it, even though these are little wider than was at first feared.

C.V. Prowse:

There is a problem in the definition of the terms. If we talk about something that is called six-hour plasma, in some centres that may be half-
an-hour old. As I understand it from Smith's data, he may have some
preliminary evidence that if it is less than four hours old it is better
than if it is less than six. And that is part of the reason that we have
been doing these experiments with the different concentrations of citrate.
If you can hold things as they are for three times as long, you may
begin to see benefits which you cannot see at the moment, because it
takes that long to get the blood to the processors. An alternative
approach to that is the freezing of plasma in the donor suite, where at
least the plasma in fresh and in your hands. It is not a nice thing to
have a huge liquid nitrogen blast freezer right next to your donor bed
in order to get it frozen within half-an-hour of donation. But you need
something along those lines in order to examine this kind of question.

J.A. Loos:

Dr. Smith, in relation to double spinning, you mentioned that it did not
influence the FVIII recovery. But did it influence the solubility of the
final cryo? If you look at the platelet contamination after a first spin in
our hands, it will be about 5 to 10% of platelets which are still present
in plasma. This is about 5×10^7 platelets ending up finally in the cryoprecipitate if you do not use a second spin. If you do the double spin,
you reduce it to about 0.5×10^7.

We saw a considerable influence, for instance, on the cloudiness of
the final preparation after solution in the buffer of the cryoprecipitate.
Did you see the same thing?

J.K. Smith:

The data I showed were rather old, and in fact obtained before the
present method for fractionation of FVIII had been developed. The data
related to source plasma and primary cryoprecipitate made in single
donations.

We have tried to keep a close eye on platelet contamination in particular. Within the limits which are followed by virtually every transfusion centre for efficient single spinning, we have not seen big
differences in the effect of platelet contamination on product. There is
one exception where one centre was not spinning very efficiently,
perhaps was taking over a little too much plasma. I should also say
that in England, the standard plasma donation is only 160 to 180 ml
instead of 250 elsewhere. So separation efficiency also has something to
do with it, not just the spinning. We have seen one case where serious
contamination of the plasma, as evidenced by red cells, as well as platelet
products, did seem to affect the stability and solubility of the concentrate during and after processing, but did not, in fact, tend to affect
the FVIII yield.

C.V. Prowse:

It is a bit disappointing to me that, as far as I can read there are no
clear statements in the literature as yet following the work in Groningen,

that heparinized plasma may run into problems when you upscale to the sort of 100 litre scale. I wonder if anybody in the audience would like to comment on their experience, should they have any of such plasma on the large scale? I understand that the Swiss Red Cross has some experience of this (3).

P. Das (Groningen):

Dr. Smith, did you consider in your presentation: a) concentration effect, b) an activated product, c) eventual instability because you are getting an activated product.

J.K. Smith:

If we had activated FVIII, we would find a very low yield in the ultimate product, which of course takes several hours to process, and then of course several days to freeze-dry. We would be most unlikely to see any benefit from activated FVIII in the concentrate; quite the opposite, you would expect to see a diminution in yield if we activated FVIII. We attribute the short NAPTT times in the Factor IX concentrate more to a probable consequence of slightly higher cell contamination. We see no reason to expect that it comes from poorer anticoagulation. In fact, you would expect that the anticoagulant would be much more efficient in the machine plasmapheresis where the anticoagulant is mixed very rapidly with the blood immediately as it leaves the vein.

I cannot explain the higher mass of cryoprecipitate. Maybe it has something to do with our particular thawing conditions. There are other differences between the standard plasma and apheresis plasma, in particular in the speed at which it is frozen. It is frozen almost immediately after donation, whereas standard plasma is frozen some 6 to 8 hours afterwards.

C.V. Prowse:

There is a pick up on one point: If this is the kind of plasma that leads to 15 to 1 anticoagulant ratio, you would expect a 10% increase in the total plasma protein, just in terms of the different ratio of anticoagulant to standard. This is my estimate, anyway.

J. Over:

Dr. Prowse, this is perhaps a difficult issue, although I do not exclude the possibility that mixing does not seem to be important for FVIII levels and the quality of FVIII, nor does the generation of FpA. You are relying on the FVIII assay by one stage or two stage? I wonder if you have ever considered the possibility of developing a test on what we would call "nativity" of FVIII. Perhaps you should compare one and two-stage assays in the same study.

C.V. Prowse:

We do that on our final products. They usually agree.

3. Morgenthaler JJ, Zuber T, Friedi H. Influence of heparin and sodium chloride on assay, stability and recovery of factor VIII. Vox Sang 1985;48:8-17.

II. Technology of plasma fractionation

SMALL POOL VERSUS LARGE POOL IN PLASMA FRACTIONATION:
REEVALUATION OF A CONCEPT

C.Th. Smit Sibinga and P.C. Das

INTRODUCTION

The concept of pool size originates from the early days of plasma
fractionation, driven by the rapidly increasing demands for plasma
protein fractions. The developments in plasma fractionation technology
have taken place much more dynamically as compared to the technical
developments in routine bloodbanking. Pharmaceutical industries have
pushed these developments to a level at which plasma fractionation could
become an independant profession, operating in a highly efficient,
scientific, technical and economical way through national or international
organisations.

NATIONAL RESOURCE

Blood is a national resource, abundantly available in each society. The
community has the moral obligation to guarantee the availability and
therefore should be regarded as the basic shareholder of the national
resource. The medical profession has the duty to protect the resource
from being overexplored as well as abused in its refinement, whether
component production or plasma fractionation, and ultimate clinical
application. In this train of thinking national self-sufficiency can be
described as the ability to collect and process sufficiently the necessary
amount of source material to provide any quality product for clinical
use (1).
    Plasma as a source material for protein fractionation so far has been
neglected in its value by Blood Banks and clinicians. Therefore, the
protein fractionation industry, both non-for-profit and commercial, have
developed systems to guarantee a minimum acceptable amount of plasma
to be collected through either "plasma campaigns" or organised plasmapheresis centres. The first route, chosen by for instance the Swiss and
Dutch Red Cross, is a simple but morally not very acceptable way of
collecting plasma. Whole blood donations are on purpose used for ex-
clusive plasma harvesting, thereby willingly wasting the cellular components. On the other hand, the plasmapheresis centres have been
organised on an almost exclusively commercial basis remunerating donors
with money, extra bonuses or a credit voucher system. Both approaches
carry major ethical objections, when compared with the fundamental
concept of altruism.

PLASMA LOGISTICS

Analysing plasma logistics, the following principles can be set:
1. Each whole blood donation comprised a plasma donation; here Blood
   Banks do have a principle responsibility.

2. Each whole blood or plasma transfusion comprises a plasma decision; a primary responsibility of the clinician.

The need for plasma is complex and depends on:
1. Clinical indications for specific proteins.
2. Plasma decisions to be made by both blood bankers and clinicians.
3. Quality assurance of the starting material, whether whole blood or plasma, because of the inevitable quantitative and qualitative losses during processing and fractionation.
4. Developments to be encouraged and implemented in processing and fractionation technology.

So, plasma, logistics depend primarily on the conceptual attitude and technical developments in both blood banking, clinical medicine and plasma fractionation.

POOL SIZE

In collection, processing and plasma fractionation, pool size is defined by the number of individual donors having contributed to the starting volume of plasma for eventual processing. In this concept WHO has given an opinion on the limit of what a small pool should be (2). This limit is based on technical possibilities and GMP restrictions within Blood Banks as practised in the 1970's. Up to twelve donations is regarded to be small pool and consequently the limit of processing within Blood Banks as related to safety, purity and potency of any final product. This concept needs reevaluation, as Blood Banks are rapidly developing their technical and processing abilities according to GMP rules. Supposedly, large pool starts at 13 donors contributing to the volume for further processing. There has never been defined an upper limit. However, a number of considerations is to be made with respect to pool size restriction, when the starting point is believed to be in the safety, purity, potency and eventual clinical efficacy of the finished product to be used:
1. Source material: Collection of plasma from whole blood donation limits the possibilities for creating small pools of considerable volume, both through the limited amount of plasma per donation and the time intervals allotted between whole blood donations. Collection of plasma by apheresis yield roughly twice the volume per donation and allows the donor to contribute to the pool more than once within a given time frame of for instance three months. The processing and storage conditions do differ between the two approaches and eventually therefore contribute to the quality of finished products.
2. Technical aspects; as conventional ethanol fractionation methodology has dominated fractionation technology, pool sizes so far were dependant on limitations of batch operation. Routinely, this approach has created much more restriction on the lower limit of the pool size, rather than on a maximum scale.
3. Economical and market conditions; the unavoidable losses in functional proteins like Factor VIII and albumin, have lead to increasing pool volumes and consequently contributing number of donors. The increasing demand created by the initial offer of purified protein fractions at good potency and expected advantages in clinical efficacy, has urged fractionators to scale up their operations, increase in pool size being a logical consequence.

LIMITING CONSEQUENCES

The lead of industry both on the collection through well organised plasmapheresis centres and the highly effective and technically well developed processing operations has further stimulated the non-for-profit sector to follow the pool size trend in its seemingly unlimited growth. However, the increasing confrontation with transmissible diseases and their strong relationship to the number of donors, contributing to the pool, has not only caused anxiety, but has urged a reevaluation of the pool size concept. Additionally, the ethanol technology has resulted in a number of physical-chemical changes of proteins such that both safety and clinical efficacy have been limiting factors in the eventual use of protein fractions. Recent developments in fractionation technology, promoted through the need for reducing losses of finished purified protein fractions, have shed new light on the possibilities for decreasing pool sizes and volumes.

REEVALUATION

As today should be regarded as tomorrow's yesterday and the future implicates both the implementation of yesterday's developments and the testing and judgment of today's innovative ideas, these possibilities need to be seriously considered and studied. The energetic and professional developments in blood banking both technical, operational and economical, which have taken place over the past decade, have opened possibilities for introduction of fractionation methodology to be operated at small scale level. Both gel column chromatography (3) controlled pore glass chromatography (4) and heparin double cold precipitation (5) principles have been introduced at Blood Bank level recently.

Gel column chromatography is practised using small pools for the production of albumin, IV-gammaglobulin and prothrombin complex concentrates. The technique is simple, needs only limited space and can be done without affecting GMP-principles at Blood Bank level. The finished protein fractions are obtained at siginificantly higher yields and better purities as compared to the classical ethanol methodology. Both the controlled pore glass chromatography and the heparin double cold precipitation method have major advantages in the production of purified Factor VIII. Small pools are extremely useful for the method, where the losses have been reduced to such an extent that self-sufficiency in this respect is within the reach of each community, even at an existing situation of still limited accessibility of this national resource.

GMP-rules have been shown to be practicable without major impact on purity or potency aspects of the most important plasma protein fractions. Safety undoubtedly will increase as the risk for transmission of diseases depends, despite all other precautions to be taken, very much on the incidence of the contamination of the pool. The greater the number of contributing donors, the higher the risk for contaminating the pool. Running costs sofar have been shown to be economically fully acceptable, both with whole blood and plasma donations as a starting material, due to the avoidance of dissipation.

Losses have been reduced, yields increased in favour of decreased risk of infection and an increase in clinical safety and efficacy. However, the smaller the volume of the pool, the greater will be the effect of the necessary sampling for quality control on the ultimate recovery of proteins. Therefore, a balance needs to be found between pool size, volumes to be processed and recoveries of purified proteins for direct clinical use, without affecting the principle of quality control.

In conclusion, reevaluation of the pool size concept, entering the fast noman's land between twelve and many, might add an entirely new dimension to the principle of national self-sufficiency: Strength through combined regional rather than a self-sustaining national effect.

REFERENCES

1. Socio-economic aspects of blood transfusion. Vox Sang 1983;44: 328-32.
2. WHO Technical Report Series 626, Geneva 1978.
3. Damevska O, Ivanovski D. Dejanov I, Kolevski P. Preparation and use of human albumin produced by large scale chromatography. Abstracts of the 18th congress of the ISBT, S. Karger Basel 1984:158.
4. Margolis J, Gallovich CM, Rhoades P. A process for preparation of 'high-purity' Factor VIII by controlled pore glass treatment. Vox Sang 1984;46:341-8.
5. Smit Sibinga CTh, Das PC. Heparin and Factor VIII. Scand J Haemat 1984;33 (suppl. 40):111-22.

ETHANOL FRACTIONATION OF HUMAN PLASMA: AN OVERVIEW

H.G.J. Brummelhuis

Human plasma is an extraordinarily complex aqueous solution of proteins, hormones, lipoids, carbohydrates etc., from which certain proteins are of interest in therapy. At the moment a small but increasing number of the hundreds of plasma proteins are used in clinical medicine and have to be prepared by fractionation. The methods applied in fractionation are more or less the same as for purification of proteins, but the aim is quite different; fractionation is meant to make the most out of plasma in terms of the clinical efficacy of the wanted protein(s). The safety of the preparations must be guaranteed by avoiding possible changes in the native structure of the protein(s) or contamination that causes side effects. The economics of fractionation also have to be considered. To reach this aim, good recovery and efficacy of the protein(s) are necessary and are mainly dependent on controlled methods and technology. The safety is dependent mainly on a correct interpretation of "Good Manufacturing Practices", which primarily is to be found in well instructed and well educated personnel, adequate housing, sanitation and equipment. Continuous attention is needed to control the costs.

During the last forty years a number of methods have been tried and performed in the fractionation of human plasma based on:
- differential solubility
- differential interaction with solid media
- differential interaction with physical fields.

For the preparation of the bulk plasma proteins, i.e. fibrinogen, immunoglobulin and albumin, the cold ethanol method, based on different solubility is generally practised although other methods based on different solubility are or have been used like fractionation with ammonium sulphate (1) and ether(2).

The separation between the proteins is performed under conditions where either the solubility of the desired protein is maximized and the solubility of the other proteins is minimized or reversed. The precipitate is separated from the supernatant by semi-continuous centrifugation and if needed, clarification.

Variables determining the precipitation of the protein(s) are:
- ethanol concentration
- pH
- temperature
- ionic strength
- protein concentration

from which the last two are less critical than the other variables and therefore mostly left out of the fractionation schemes. The first large scale batchwise fractionation of human plasma using acetate buffers was described by Cohn and coworkers who developed a number of methods from which the method 5 and 6 (3) and the immunoglobulin method 9 according to Oncley et al. (4) are the best known.

In the flowsheet (fig. 1) other products like plasminogen, prothrombin complex etc., which can be prepared from fraction II+III and a further purification of fraction II has been left out. By this combined method five preparations can be derived from human plasma:

48

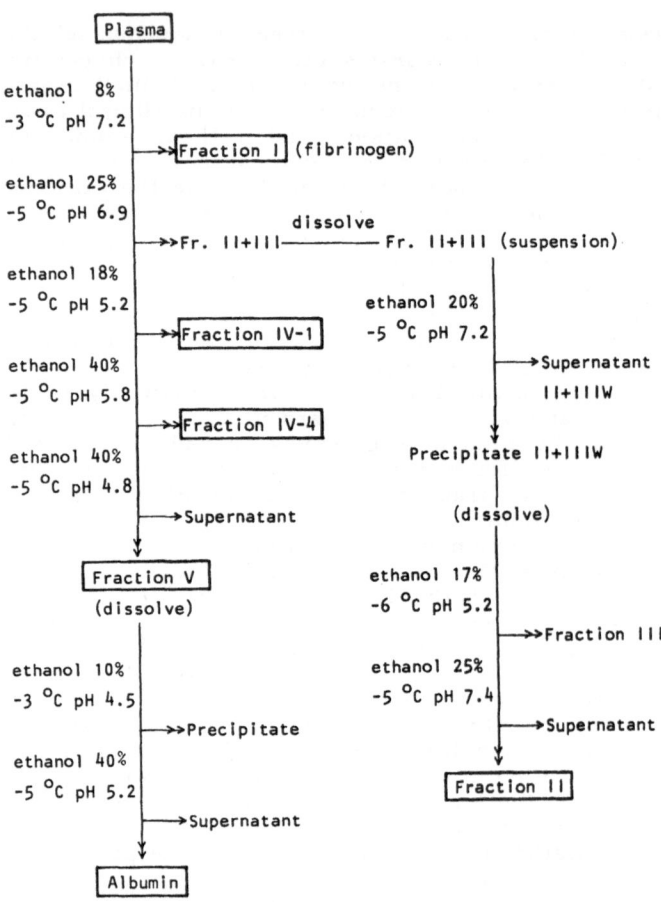

Figure 1. Flowsheet for the preparation of the bulk plasma derivatives according to Cohn, Oncley and coworkers

Fraction I as fibrinogen
Fraction II as immunoglobulin
Fraction IV-4 and V as pasteurized plasma protein fraction (PPF; 85% albumin)
Fraction V as pasteurized plasma protein fraction (PPF; 90% albumin) and Albumin (>96% albumin).

After the introduction of this fractionation method a number of investigators have introduced modifications to simplify the method, especially in Europe, to achieve higher recoveries, equal or even better safety and efficacy and lower costs. During and after World War II Mastenbroek (the Netherlands) started cold ethanol fractionation of human plasma using sodium hydroxide and citric acid instead of acetate buffers for fixing the pH. This resulted in the following method of fractionation (5). By method described in the flowsheet (fig. 2) four preparations, fibrinogen, immunoglobulin, PPF (90% albumin) and Albumin (>96% albumin) can be prepared but by a much easier way than those of Cohn and Oncley. Also Kistler and Nitschmann(6) of the Swiss Red Cross Blood Transfusion Service introduced a modified and easier method, using acetate buffers and different ethanol concentrations and temperatures (fig. 3).

Other fractionation centres modify or have modified the cold ethanol method by introducing other principles of separation like adsorbents as by Björling at KABI, Sweden (7). For further purification of fraction II to almost pure IgG (>98%) an adsorption step to DEAE Sephadex A-50 has been performed. To increase the recovery of the albumin, fraction IV is precipitated at a concentration of 35% ethanol and not at 40%. The so recovered fraction V is less pure, but adsorption to C.M. Sephadex C-50 allows the standard of purity to be reached.

Although Cohn et al. (3) first introduced the use of diatomaceous earth for clarification of supernatants after semi-continuous centrifugation, fractionation centres also developed the filtration with filteraids instead of semi-continuous centrifugation, as a saving of time and energy as first published by Friedli et al (8).

A number of centres do not use all the plasma for the preparation of fibrinogen and immunoglobulin. To increase the fractionation capacity and decrease costs, some introduced the precipitation of fraction I-III or I-IV in one step. Others introduced a combination of ethanol fractionation and heating in the presence of caprylate (9, 10).

The cold ethanol method is mostly performed as a batchwise (300-5,000 1) process. A number of complicating factors like heat transfer and effective mixing can better be handled in small volumes than in large volumes. However, the small volume treatment could not be performed without disturbing the fractionation capacity. To overcome these problems and since automatic process control systems have been developed, a continuous flow instead of a batchwise process is possible and has been introduced by Watt (11) at the Scottish National Blood Transfusion Service in Edinburgh.

The fractionation methods mentioned till now are used for human plasma. The cold ethanol method has served also as backbone of the fractionation of placental extract. For this fractionation a number of extra steps have to be introduced for an almost complete removal of bloodgroup substances, tissue antigens, haemderivatives etc. The preparation of albumin according to Liautaud (12) has been taken for an exemple (fig. 4). Later on, Tayot et al. (13) simplified this extended procedure by adsorption of dissolved fraction V to Spherosil-DEAE Dextran.

50

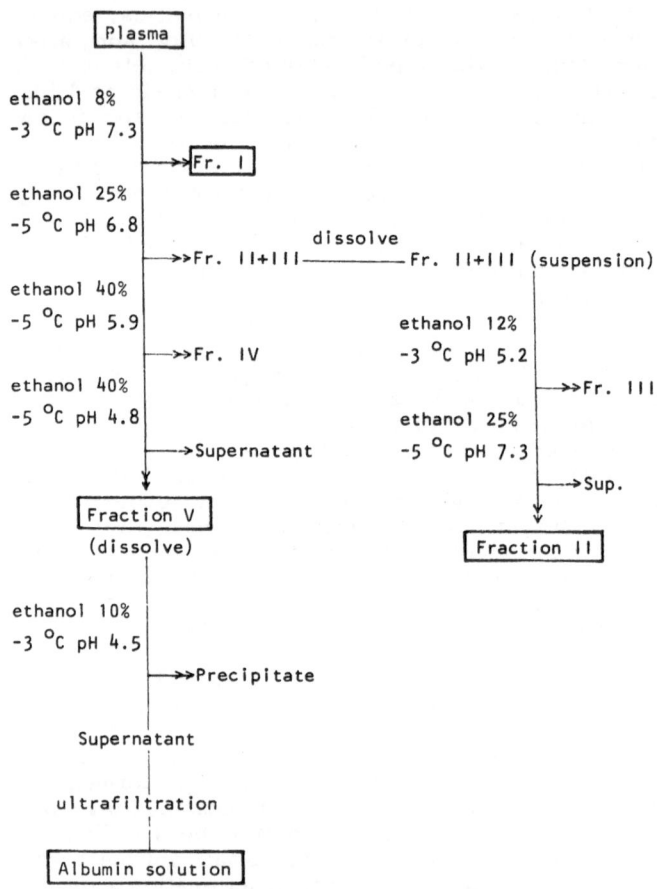

Figure 2. Flowsheet for the preparation of the bulk plasma
derivatives as performed by the Central Laboratory of the
Netherlands Red Cross Blood Transfusion Service

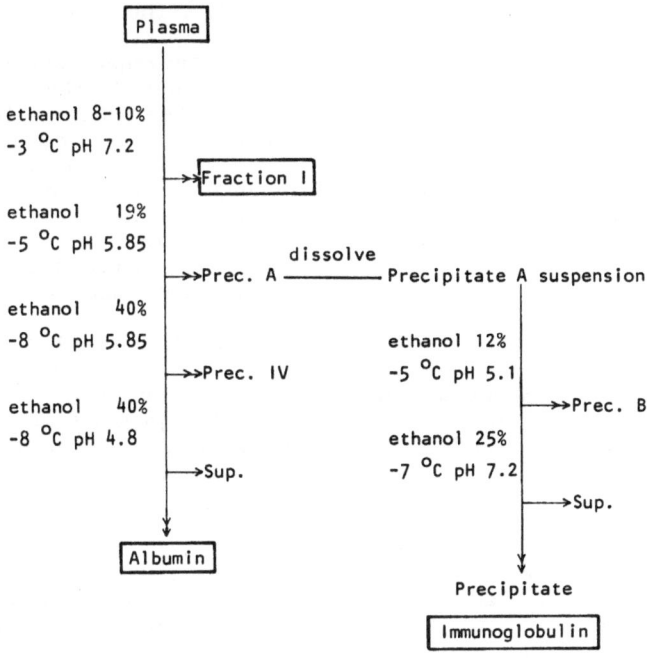

Figure 3. Flowsheet for the preparation of the bulk plasma
derivatives as performed by the Swiss Red Cross Blood
Transfusion Service

For the preparation of specific immunoglobulin, the normal plasma has to be replaced by specific plasma. This specific plasma has to contain about one tenth of the wanted strength of the final specific immunoglobulin. In the fractionation of specific plasma the division of the immunoglobulin over fraction II and III is mostly analogous with the division of the specific antibodies with exception of anti-D which possesses a lower recovery in fraction II (14).

During the final processing of Fraction II, the immunoglobulin and the traces of contaminating other proteins are partially modified with the consequence that the immunoglobulin cannot be injected intravenously without side effects like anaphylactoid reactions which are related to certain IgG aggregates. Furthermore vasoactive reactions occur which are related to activated components e.g. clotting factor XIIa (PKA) and the so-called phlogistic reactions related to physiological antigen-antibody reactions. This last type of reactions can only be induced with intact antibodies and not with fragmented IgG like Fab and $F(ab')_2$ and is in reality a good criterion of the efficacy i.e. the native state of the immunoglobulin preparation (15).

For the preparation of immunoglobulin for intravenous administration, most fractionation centres start with Cohn fraction II. Cohn fraction II is either treated with enzymes like pepsin and plasmin to $F(ab')_2$ respectively (partially) Fab fragmentation of IgG3 and IgG1 (the complement related IgG's), or with chemicals like β-propiolacton and reducing agents of immunoglobulin or physical treatment, like pH with a trace of pepsin, further purification with adsorbents or ion exchangers or combinations of those (16). At the moment the physically treated immunoglobulin preparations are preferred, especially the ones that posses the same subclass distribution of IgG as normal human plasma (17, 18).

As shown, most of the fractionation methods finish with a precipitate containing ethanol. The precipitate has to be dissolved and further processed to give a product that can be stored and can be injected in humans. For removing ethanol and bringing the product in the desired concentration, three methods or combinations of that are possible.

FREEZE-DRYING(19)

The principle of freeze-drying is based on the removal of volatile components i.e. water and ethanol from the solid state directly to the vapour state at low pressure. In freeze-drying three stages are discerned: the freezing, the primary drying i.e. sublimation of ice and the secondary drying i.e. desorption of water. Although the principle of the process is simple, the control of the factors influencing the quality of the product requires a good understanding of all the details of the process and a rather complicated and expensive equipment. In the past the correct conditions have been found by trial and error, but the understanding of the principles of the freezing and drying characteristics is still increasing permitting gradually replacement of the trial and error method. The knowledge and equipment is still needed for the preparations of human plasma, that have to be stored in the lyophilized state. For the preparation that can be stored in the liquid state, other ways are possible and in case of albumin preferred.

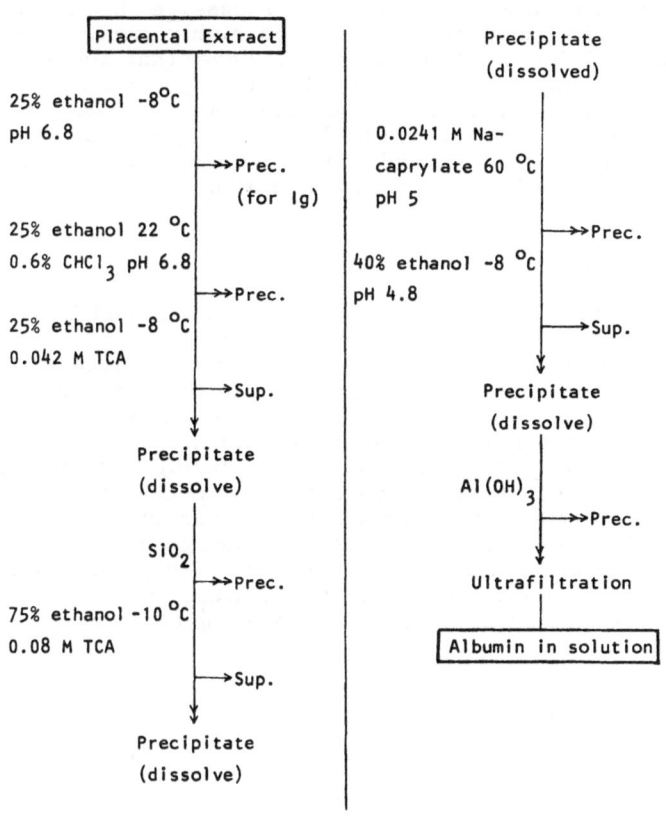

Figure 4. Flowsheet for the preparation of placental albumin
as performed by Institute Mérieux, France

SEPARATION BY FILTRATION BASED ON DIFFERENCE OF MOLECULAR SIZES

For the removal of low molecular weight components like salts and ethanol from high molecular components (proteins) two systems are now practised.

Gelfiltration (20)

The molecules in solution can enter to varying extent into the swollen gelbeads depending on their size and shape. If the molecules are larger than the largest pores in the swollen gel bed, they do not enter while the other molecules are retarded by their passage through the gel bed. The procedure can easily be performed on highly cross-linked, hardgels like Sephadex G-25, on large scale provided that the equipment has been automated and a reliable supply of large amounts of water for injection can be generated. The procedure does not harm the proteins if the gelfiltration has been performed under appropriate conditions like germ-free or germ-poor (< 100/ml) circumstances. After gelfiltration, the solution may be concentrated by ultrafiltration.

Ultrafiltration (21)

In case of ultrafiltration – mostly diafiltration, followed by ultrafiltration – the dissolved molecules are separated by passing or not-passing a selective permeable membrane. Molecules above a nominal size and shape are retarded while below that shape and size they can pass through the membrane under pressure. A number of variables are important like pH, concentration, temperature, since these influence the size and shape of the molecule and therefore the separation. During ultrafiltration another phenomenon starts, namely concentration polarization, that is the formation on the membrane surface of a layer of concentrated macromolecules. This concentration of macromolecules reduces the flow and alters the retention characteristics. To reduce this phenomenon agitation and if possible increasing the temperature is introduced. Under appropriate condition this procedure is very gentle and does no or little harm to the product.

THIN FILM EVAPORATION (22)

In contrast to freeze-drying, volatile components are removed from a solution bringing the volatile components from the fluid to the vapour state under vacuum. In this process the solution is spread over a supporting surface to which heat is applied. Under this condition ethanol and a certain part of the water is removed while the proteins and the salts are remaining in the solution. This method has to be restricted to albuminoid solutions, that have already a low salt content and contain stabilizers like caprylate. The procedure has to be strictly controlled, since failure like for example prolonged exposure to heat do harm the albumin. After removal of the unwanted components, the preparation is brought in its final composition (clarified), sterile filtered and dispensed in ampoules or bottles and closed. The fibrinogen is freeze-dried, the normal immunoglobulin is in solution, while the albuminoid solutions are pasteurized for 10-11 hours at 60 ± 0.5°C. The final product has to pass the quality control and must meet the requirements prescribed by the Health Authorities. Thereafter the product can be distributed.

The past has proven, that the cold ethanol method has met and can meet in a reasonable way the aim of fractionation namely high recovery, maintained efficacy, safety and low costs of the bulk plasma derivatives. Taking into account the trace components (clotting factors VIII, IX, antithrombin III, etc.) also, plasma fractionation has already been extended with other methodologies and is not any more restricted to cold ethanol fractionation. It must be clear, that certain aspects of fractionation like modifications in methodology e.g. combination with other methods based on other principles, in technology e.g. more detailed process control and in equipment e.g. larger scale and more closed systems in final processing can be improved and thus can contribute to meet the aim of fractionation in a better way.

REFERENCES

1. Schwick HG. A survey of the production of plasmaderivatives for clinical use. Vox Sang 1972;23:82.
2. Keckwick. RA. Medical Research Council Report Series No. 286. Her Majesty's Stationary Office 1954.
3. Cohn EJ, Strong LE, Hughes Jr WJ et al. Preparation and properties of serum and plasmaproteins IV. A system for the preparation into fractions of the protein and lipoprotein components of biological tissues and fluids. J Am Chem Soc 1946;68:459-75.
4. Oncley JL. Melin M, Richert DA, Cameron JW, Gross Jr PM. The separation of the antibodies, isoagglutinins, prothrombin, plasminogen and β_1-lipoprotein into subfractions of human plasma. J Am Chem Soc 1949;71:541-50.
5. Brummelhuis, HGJ. Techniques in use for plasma fractionation. Acta Pharm Suec 1983;4:91-97.
6. Kostler P, Nitschmann H. Large scale production of human plasma fractions. Vox Sang 1962;7:414-24.
7. Björling H. Industrial plasma fractionation methods. In: Blombäck B, Hanson LA, eds. Plasma Proteins. Chicester: John Wiley and Sons, 1979:29-37.
8. Friedli H, Mauerhofer M, Faes A, Kistler P. Studies on new process procedures in plasma fractionation on an industrial scale. Vox Sang 1976;31:289-95.
9. Schneider W, Lefevre H, Friedler H, McCarthy LJ. An alternative method of large scale plasma fractionation for the isolation of serum albumin. Blut 1975;30:131-4.
10. Villiers V, Wilson JGS. Ethanol and heat-treated plasma fractionation methods in South Africa. Vox Sang 1978;35:48-9.
11. Watt JG. Automatic fractionation of plasma proteins. Vox Sang 1972;23:126-34.
12. Liautaud J, Pla J, Debrus A, Gattel P, Plan R, Peyron L. Préparation de l'albumine humaine à partir de sang hémolysé extrait de placentas congelés. I. Technique de préparation et qualité du produit. Develop Biol Standard 1974;27:107-14.
13. Tayot JL, Tardy M, Gattel P. Ion exchange and affinity chromatography on silica derivatives. In: Curling JM, ed. Methods of Plasma Protein Fractionation. London: Academic Press Inc. 1980:149-60.
14. Vogelaar EF, Boer-vd Berg MAG de, Burmmelhuis HGJ, Beentjes SP, Krijnen HW. Contributions to the optimal use of human blood. IV. Quantitative analysis of the immunoglobulin isolation. Vox Sang 1974;27:193-206.

15. Barandun S, Morell A, Skvaril F. Clinical experiences with immunoglobulin for intravenous use. In: Alving BM, Finlayson JS, ed. Immunoglobulins, characteristics and uses of intravenous preparations. DHHS Publication No. (FDA)80-9005. U.S. Dept of Health and Human Services 1979:31-5.
16. Finlayson JS, Alving BM. Overview of potential uses for immunoglobulin preparations, possible etiologies of adverse reactions and ideal characteristics of intravenous preparations. In: Alving BM, Finlayson JS, ed. Immunoglobulins, characteristics and uses of intravenous preparations. DHHS Publication No. (FDA)80-9005. U.S. Dept. of Healt and Human Services 1979:229-34.
17. Römer J, Morgenthaler JJ, Scherz R, Skvaril F, Characterization of various immunoglobulin preparations for intravenous application I. Vox Sang 1982;42:62-73.
18. Piët MPJ, Moors JJP, Niessen JCM, Schellekens PThA, Brummelhuis HGJ. Bereiding, karakterisering en klinisch gebruik van een immunoglobuline preparaat voor intraveneuze toepassing. Pharm Weekbl 1984;119:700-7.
19. MacKenzie AP. Solvent exchange and removal-lyophilization. In: Sandberg HE, ed. Proc Int Workshop on Technology for Protein Separation and Improvement of Blood Plasma Fractionation. DHEW Publication No. (NIH)78-1422. Dept. of Health, Education and Welfare 1978:245-8.
20. Friedli H. Kistler P. Removal of ethanol from albumin by gelfiltration in the manufacturing of human serum albumin solutions for clinical use. Chimia 1972;26:25-7.
21. Martinache L, Henon MP. Concentration and desalting by ultrafiltration. In: Curling JM, ed. Methods of Plasma Protein Fractionation. London: Academic Press Inc. 1980:223-34.
22. Vallet L. Thin film evaporation for the removal of solvents. In: Curling JL, ed. Methods of Plasma Protein Fractionation. London: Academic Press Inc. 1980:211-22.

CONTROL OF LARGE-SCALE PLASMA THAWING

P.R. Foster, and A.J. Dickson

INTRODUCTION

The freezing and thawing of plasma is an essential part of plasma fractionation when carried out as an industrial pharmaceutical manufacturing operation. Consequently the manner in which these procedures are carried out can have a major impact on the yield and quality of products, plant capacity and process logistics. This is particularly true of factor VIII manufacture where the labile protein is initially extracted from cryoprecipitate formed during the freeze-thaw process.

Cryoprecipitation is a convenient and useful step which is used in virtually all methods of factor VIII production, however it is this step which is primarily responsible for the low yields characteristic of industrial-scale processing (1).

Loss of factor VIII is probably due to a number of mechanisms. It is recognised that protein can be damaged by the high concentrations of salts and extremes of pH which form within the frozen mass when the various solutes become mobile (2). This occurs between the eutectic and melting point temperatures but is generally considered to be most severe in the range -8°C to -3°C as it is in this region that solutes are both sufficiently mobile and concentrated to cause maximum damage (3). Attack by proteolytic enzymes (4) is also likely to occur at the same time.

The degree of damage by these mechanisms can be minimised by thawing rapidly but this introduces a further problem. The solubility of cryoprecipitated factor VIII is strongly temperature dependent and, although the exact relationship has not yet been fully determined, it is clear that local overshooting of temperature during thawing will cause precipitated factor VIII to go back into solution to be lost into the cryosupernatant (5).

To resolve these various problems it has been necessary to design a method of thawing which is both rapid and free from temperature overshoot. This has been achieved by thawing crushed frozen plasma in a continuous manner whereby plasma is removed from the source of heating as soon as the liquid phase forms. The design and operation of this process has been previously reported (5), our further experiences with this method will be described here.

THE OVERALL THAWING PROCESS

Prior to fractionation plasma is held in cold storage at -40°C and, from the reasoning above, our initial objective was to take this plasma to 0°C as rapidly as possible. Although the continuous crush-thaw process was capable of doing this, we discovered that this procedure gave a poor yield of factor VIII in a cryoprecipitate which was particularly difficult to process (5). In contrast, high yields of Factor VIII were achieved when the rapid crush-thaw process was used only over the latter phase of thawing (ie -10°C to 0°C).

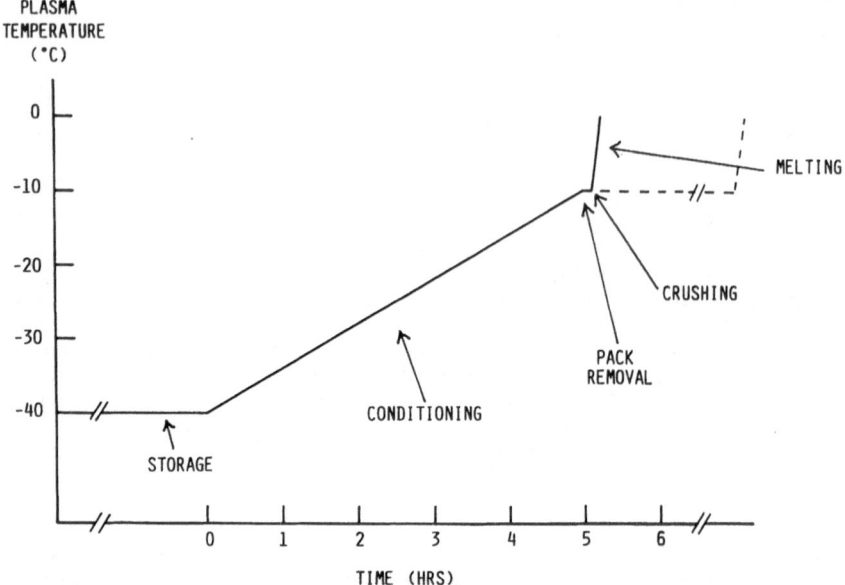

Figure 1. Schematic representation of the present Scottish procedure for thawing plasma.

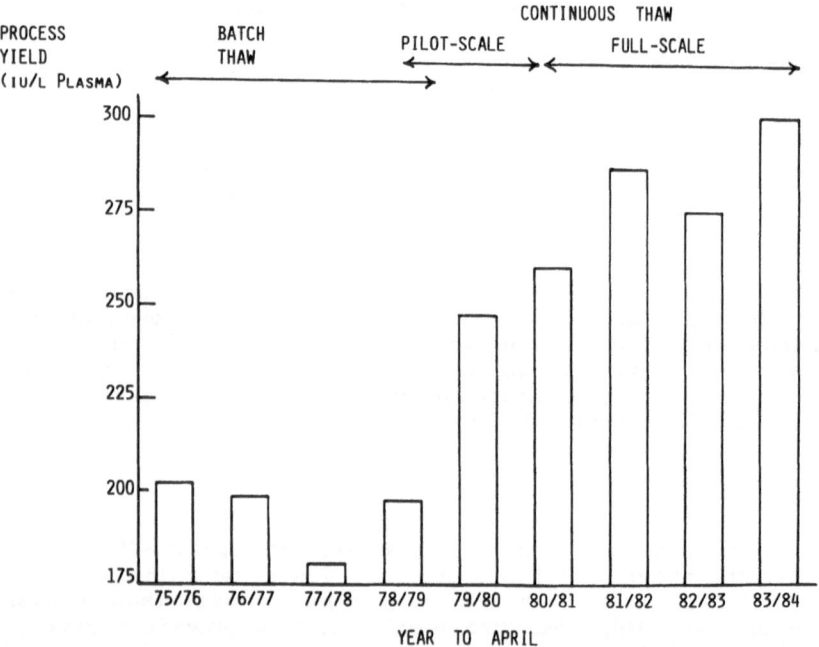

Figure 2. Process yield of intermediate-purity factor VIII concentrate from 1975-1984.

The overall procedure (fig. 1) now involves four distinct phases each of which must be carefully designed and controlled to maximise factor VIII yield.

1. Conditioning. The relatively slow warming of frozen plasma from −40°C to about −10°C over about 5 hours is needed to form a readily soluble cryoprecipitate which aids further processing. This has been traditionally done by holding the plasme in a +4°C room. More regular and precise performance is achieved using a small unit with a high velocity air-stream to achieve the desired temperature according to a selected control program.

2. Pack Removal. Removal of the plasma container is ideally integrated into the process following the conditioning phase. This avoids the need to impose further temperature perturbations on the plasma (eg by returning to −40°C) and enables the container to be removed at a point when the plastic is flexible and easily separated from the plasma. A manual cutting procedure is normally employed but this may be both dangerous (6) and dirty, providing a route for the transfer of bacteria from the outer surface of the container into the plasma stream (7). An automated method is therefore highly desirable and attempts to deal with the problem in this way are in progress using either cutting (8) or tearing (9) actions.

3. Crushing. A high surface area of frozen plasma is essential if a high rate of heat transfer is to be obtained. This can be achieved by crushing the frozen individual plasma donations into small particles. The plasma snow produced in this way is also capable of being mixed by an agitator, which further aids heat transfer and keeps the melted liquid in contact with frozen material to maintain a low temperature in the fluid phase.

4. Melting. This final phase of the thawing process involves the rapid thawing of the crushed plasma ice to the liquid state. A continuous process has been designed for this purpose utilising a stirred, heated vessel of about 55 litres volume (5).

CONTINUOUS MELTING

1. Operational Performance

The capacity or throughput of the continuous-thaw apparatus is proportional to the area of heated vessel wall, while the plasma temperature is controlled by mixing at the wall using a double helical ribbon agitator (10) and by continuous removal of the liquid phase by gravity via a weir arrangement. The apparatus was designed on this basis to operate with a throughput of about 200 kg plasma per hour with the plasma temperature held below +2°C at the warmest point at the vessel wall (5).

Monitoring of the plasma film temperature has shown that at the warmest point the temperature remains close to 0°C from start-up to shut-down of the process (11) and mean data from a number of consecutive lots (table 1) indicates that this performance is achieved routinely. Although the temperature of the plasma leaving the thawing vessel is consistently below 0°C a crush-thaw rate of about 200 kg/hr is sustained (table 1).

This careful control is essential for the efficient preparation of factor VIII from fresh frozen plasma however the crush-thaw equipment is also applicable to the processing of time-expired or hyperimmune plasmas. In this instance the temperature of the water-jacket heating the vessel can be raised from 22°C (used for fresh plasma) to 32°C giving a thaw rate of about 280 kg/hr with the plasma film temperature still below +4°C and the plasma outlet temperature below +1°C.

2. Cryoprecipitate Composition

Fresh frozen plasma is received from Transfusion Centres in Scotland and Northern Ireland categorised as 6 hour plasma or 18 hour plasma according to the delay between the time of donation and the time of freezing for cold-storage. At the Fractionation Centre the pool size for continuous thawing is currently either 600 kg or 1000 kg plasma according to the size of freeze drier available.

Some characteristics of continuous-thaw cryoprecipitate produced from 20 recent, consecutive, 1000 kg plasma production lots are listed in table 2 alongside details of 20 consecutive batch thaw lots. Similar data are shown for 12 lots of 18 hour plasma in table 3. There is a 51% increase in FVIII recovery from the continuous crush-thaw procedure for 6 hour plasma and a 33% increase for 18 hour plasma compared to the batch process previously used. Although the % standard deviation in factor VIII recovery is similar for batch and continuous processing the % S.D. for cryoprecipitate weight and protein content are significantly lower for material processed continuously, suggesting that the procedure is much more reproducible on a lot to lot basis than the smaller volume batch process.

Comparison of 6 hour and 18 hour plasmas shows that the cryo-precipitate factor VIII recoveries from continuous thawing are similar when expressed as a % of the FVIII C monitored in the starting plasma, indicating that differences in plasma quality are reflected in the subsequent recovery of FVIII C.

The composition of cryosupernatant from the continuous-thaw process is shown in table 4 where both FVIII C and FVIII R:Ag are consistently close to the lowest level that can probably be expected from normal solubility behaviour (12). Similar data have been previously reported for FVIII C:Ag (11).

It is interesting to note that 90% of the plasma FVIII C can be accounted for in the precipitate plus supernatant suggesting that about 10% of the plasma FVIII C is still being inactivated at some point in the process.

3. Impact on Factor VIII Production

An intermediate-purity factor VIII concentrate is prepared by this extraction of cryoprecipitate, adsorption of protein contaminants with aluminium hydroxide and filtration through a 0.22 μm membrane filter (5). The overall yield of factor VIII from this process is shown in table 5 for the same lots considered above, showing a mean improvement of 44% for 6 hour plasma and 54% for 18 hour plasma from the continuous thaw process. The batch and continuous-thaw lots compared in tables 2-5 were not processed at the same time and some process details have changed in the intervening period. These include differences in plasma quality and improvements in equipment for plasma conditioning (fig. 1), mixing and centrifugation (11). These latter changes have developed from the fact that continuous-thaw cryoprecipitate has been found to be more soluble and generally easier to process than that resulting from batch thawing.

Table 1. Operational data from continuous thaw process

	6 HR PLASMA (N=20)	18 HR PLASMA (N=12)
PLASMA TEMPERATURE (°C)		
WALL FILM	0.67 ± 0.35 *	0.67 ± 0.56
OUTLET	-0.66 ± 0.54	-0.50 ± 0.58
RATE OF THAW (KG/HR)	201.4 ± 8.8	202.0 ± 14.9

* RESULTS ARE EXPRESSED AS THE MEAN ± STANDARD DEVIATION.

Table 2. Comparison of batch and continuous thaw processes (6 hour plasma)

	CONTINUOUS THAW (N=20)	BATCH THAW (N=20)
POOL SIZE (KG)	965.4 ± 39.7	160.6 ± 21.1
CRYOPRECIPITATE		
WEIGHT (G/L PLASMA)	9.04 ± 0.64	8.49 ± 1.37
PROTEIN (G/L PLASMA)	1.18 ± 0.10	1.06 ± 0.20
FVIII C (IU/L PLASMA)	479.3 ± 101.1	316.5 ± 60.4
FVIII C (% PLASMA FVIII C)	63.5	

Table 3. Comparison of batch and continuous thaw processes (18 hour plasma)

	CONTINUOUS THAW (N=12)	BATCH THAW (N=12)
POOL SIZE (KG)	980.7 ± 28.4	138.9 ± 18.3
CRYOPRECIPITATE		
WEIGHT (G/L PLASMA)	9.53 ± 1.08	8.93 ± 2.14
PROTEIN (G/L PLASMA)	1.24 ± 0.17	0.88 ± 0.32
FVIII C (IU/L PLASMA)	370.6 ± 66.8	278.2 ± 95.6
FVIII C (% PLASMA FVIII C)	60.7	

Table 4. Factor VIII remaining in cryosupernatant from continuous thaw process

	6 HR PLASMA (N=20)	18 HR PLASMA (N=12)
VIII C (IU/L PLASMA)	206 ± 74	190 ± 50
VIII C (% PLASMA VIII C)	27.3	31.1
VIII R:AG (U/L PLASMA)	150 ± 87	150 ± 140
VIII R:AG (% PLASMA VIII R:AG)	13.6	14.1

Table 5. Process yield of factor VIII (intermediate-purity concentrate)

	CONTINUOUS THAW	BATCH THAW
6 HOUR PLASMA (N=20)		
FACTOR VIII YIELD		
(IU/L PLASMA)	293.4 ± 43.0	204.1 ± 37.0
(% PLASMA FVIII)	38.9	
18 HOUR PLASMA (N=12)		
FACTOR VIII YIELD		
(IU/L PLASMA)	268.0 ± 42.3	173.8 ± 49.3
(% PLASMA FVIII)	43.9	

Table 6. Advantages of continues thaw process.

1. INCREASED YIELD OF FVIII

2. IMPROVED SOLUBILITY OF CRYOPRECIPITATE

3. EASY TO INCREASE BATCH SIZE

4. WIDE RANGE OF BATCH SIZES POSSIBLE WITH NO CHANGE IN PERFORMANCE

5. CONVENIENT FOR ALL TYPES OF PLASMA (INCLUDING TIME EXPIRED, HYPERIMMUNE)

6. EQUIPMENT IS COMPACT, RELIABLE AND SIMPLE TO OPERATE AND MAINTAIN

The overall impact of the continuous-thaw process can therefore be best appreciated from the process yield of intermediate-purity concentrate calculated for all lots processed during the last 9 years. This information is shown in fig. 2 where the overall improvement in yield from the final period batch processing (1977/78) to the present time (1983/84) has been about 65%.

Some other advantages of the continuous-thaw process are listed in table 6. In particular the change from batch to continuous processing has enabled the plasma pool size to be increased relatively easily so that a 3.7 fold increase in plasma throughput has been accomodated since 1977/78 without any major increase in staffing or facilities to handle the thawing operation.

This substantial increase in plasma throughput taken together with the significant increase in factor VIII yield has resulted in a 7-fold increase in the output of SNBTS factor VIII concentrate for clinical use (fig. 3). Hence it can be concluded that control of plasma thawing has played an important role in enabling National self-sufficiency to be achieved.

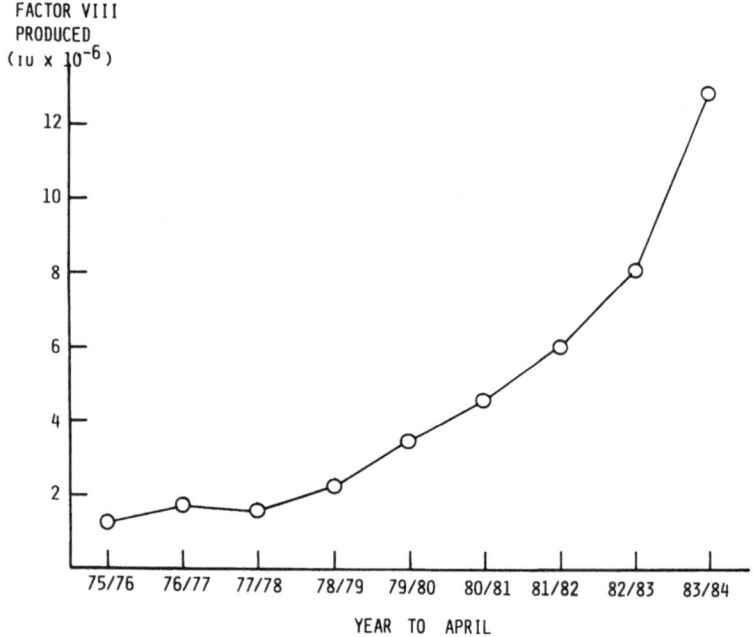

Figure 3. Production of SNBTS intermediate-purity factor VIII concentrate from 1975-1984.

REFERENCES

1. Prowse CV, Griffin B, Pepper DS, et al. Changes in factor VIII complex activities during the production of a clinical intermediate purity factor VIII concentrate. Thromb. Haemostas 1981;46:597-601.
2. Chilson OP, Costello LA, Kaplan. Effects of freezing on enzymes. Fed Proc. 1965;24:S55-S65.
3. Webb FC. Biochemical Engineering. London: Van Nostrad, 1964:362.
4. Atichartakarn V, Marder VJ, Kirby EP, Budzynski AZ. Effects of enzyme degradation on the subunit composition and biologic properties of human factor VIII. Blood 1978;51:281-97.
5. Foster PR, Dickson AJ, McQuillan TA, Dickson IH, Keddie S, Watt JG. Control of large-scale plasma thawing for recovery of cryo-precipitate factor VIII. Vox Sang. 1982;42:180-9.
6. Taylor JS, Shmunes MD, Holmes AW. Hepatitis B in plasma fractionation workers. JAMA 1974;230:850-3.
7. Watt JG, Perry RJ, Cuthbertson B. Contamination of plasma for fractionation: a design solution Lancet. 1982;i:909-10. (letter)
8. Lane RS. The single plasma pack: IPP. In: Further developments in transfusion practice. Lancaster, MTP Press, 1981:25-46.
9. Perry RJ, Cuthbertson B, Dickson AJ, Foster PR, Neillie G. Blood bag developments — a fractionators view. In: Abstracts 18th Congress ISBT. S. Karger Basel 1984:68.
10. Foster PR, Dunnill P, Lilly MD. The kinetics of protein salting-out: precipitation of yeast enzymes by ammonium sulphate. Biotech Bioeng 1976;XVIII:545-80.
11. Foster PR, Dickson AJ, Dickson IH. Improving yield in the manufacture of factor VIII concentrates. Scand. J. Haematol 1984;33,(Suppl 40):103-11.
12. Over J, Bouma BN, Van Mourik JA, Sixma JJ, Vlooswijk R, Bakker-Woudenberg I. Heterogeneity of human factor VIII. 1 characterisation of factor VIII present in the supernatant of cryo-precipitate. J. Lab Clin. Med. 1978;91:32-46.

CONTRIBUTIONS TO THE OPTIMIZATION OF FACTOR VIII PRODUCTION: CRYOPRECIPITATION AND CONTROLLED PORE GLASS ADSORPTION

J. Over, M.P.J. Piët, J.A. Loos, H.P.J. Henrichs, P.J. Hoek, M.A. von Meyenfeldt and J.I.H. Oh.

INTRODUCTION

The steadily increasing need for factor VIII complex to treat hemophilia A in an optimal way, nowadays causes a heavy demand for fresh-frozen plasma, from which this clotting factor is isolated. This is directly caused by the low recoveries of factor VIII coagulant activity (VIII:C) in most fractionation procedures, due to the lability of VIII:C as well as to the circumstance that also other plasma components are to be isolated from the plasma. Cryoprecipitation for instance usually yields recoveries of 300-500 units out of every 1000 that theoretically are present in 1 liter of starting plasma. Further purification to a high purity concentrate causes additional substantial loss. In routine practice therefore final recoveries of 100-200 IU/l are normal which means that about 80% of the potential supply of VIII:C is spoilt. Yet, cryoprecipitation is still generally applied as the first step in factor VIII production, because of the purification obtained, the simplicity of the process and the fact that the other plasma proteins can still be isolated from the cryosupernatant. Although quite some literature has appeared in the past two decades dealing with the influence of several parameters on the recovery and purity of VIII:C in cryoprecipitate (e.g. 1,2), it is still not known by what mechanism the factor VIII complex is precipitating during freezing and thawing of plasma. As more knowledge of the basic phenomena that take place during cryoprecipitation might enable a better performance of the process, the behaviour of the factor VIII complex as well as that of salt and proteins other than factor VIII was analyzed during freezing and thawing of plasma. To this end several freezing and thawing regimes were applied to bags filled with a standard volume of plasma, from which samples were drawn both during and after freezing or thawing. This approach led to the conclusion that cryoprecipitation is not a salting-out process and secondly that both the freezing and thawing process of plasma should be fast for optimal performance with regard to VIII:C.
Secondly, the application of controlled-pore glass (CPG) to prepare a high purity concentrate from cryoprecipitate was studied in an extensive way, as this technique was claimed to yield a high-purity concentrate showing VIII:C recoveries over 80% relative to cryoprecipitate (3, 4). In our study the optimal conditions were determined for the CPG adsorption after which the VIII:C-containing effluent was submitted to a concentrating step. When prepared on a laboratory scale the final product after reconstitution has an VIII:C concentration up to 40 IU/ml and a specific activity of 2-4 IU/mg. More important however, is the recovery which at present is 230 IU/l.

MATERIALS AND METHODS

Plasma.

The plasma that was used in the study consisted of a pool of ACD-plasma of 10 or 70 donations, with an VIII:C concentration of 0.75-0.95 IU/ml, which was filled into bags in 300 ml aliquots. Two types of bags were used: a smaller one of 300 ml total contents (surface area 310 m^2; Terumo Corp., Japan) and a larger one of 600 ml contents (surface area 450 cm^2; NPBI, Emmer-Compascuum, The Netherlands). When filled with 300 ml plasma the thickness of plasma was about 4 and 2 cm respectively.

Freezing conditions and sampling techniques.

For the study on freezing, four freezing regimes were applied on both types of plasma bags: a) immersion in CO_2-ethanol (-79°C), b) laying in circulating N_2-gas of -100°C, c), laying in stationary air of -30°C and d) laying in a polystyrene foam box that was put in stationary air of -30°C. This resulted in the following average freezing times (measured in the centre of the bag): a) 11 and 7 minutes respectively, b) 12 and 10 minutes, c) 4 and 3 hours and d) 19 and 15 hours.

Samples were drawn in two ways both during freezing at certain time intervals and after complete freezing. During freezing the first way consisted of drawing a 1 ml sample from the centre and the second way of drawing the total liquid remainder. After freezing the first way consisted of drawing a core sample (1.4 cm ∅) from the centre and dividing it in a top, centre and bottom part, and the second way of cutting a complete longitudinal section from the ice (2 cm wide) and dividing it in 6-8 segments of equal length.

When the influence of freezing on cryoprecipitation was assessed, thawing was performed by putting the bags in a rocking waterbath of 4°C.

Thawing conditions and sampling techniques.

For the study on thawing only the larger type of bags was used (filled with 300 ml of plasma), which were frozen in a fast as well as a slow way: immersion in CO_2-ethanol (freezing time about 10 minutes) and laying in stationary air of -30°C while placed one against another (freezing time about 4-6 h).

Both batchwise thawing and thaw-siphoning (5, 6) were applied on both types of frozen plasma. For batchwise thawing the thawing media consisted of a) a waterbath of 20°C, b) a waterbath of 4°C, and c) stationary air of 4°C, resulting in thawing times of about 15 min., 1 h and 20 h, respectively. For thaw-siphoning also several regimes were applied: waterbathes ranging in temperatures from 20°C down to 4°C and stationary air of 20°C, resulting in thawing times of 12 min. up to 45 min., and 90 min., respectively.

Samples during batchwise thawing were taken by drawing the total liquid phase at certain time intervals. In thaw-siphoning the effluent was sampled.

Analyses on plasma samples.

Plasma samples were analyzed for the following parameters:
VIII:C by one-stage assay (7, 8); total protein by the biuret method;
albumin by radial immunodiffusion (Mancini technique) in freezing study,
or by immunoturbidimetry in a Vitatron PA 800 autoanalyzer similarly
as described by Out et al. (9); IgM, IgG and IgA by immunoturbidimetry
(9); Na$^+$ by flame photometry in a semi-automated flame photometer
(model 543, Instrumentation Laboratory, Italy).

Analyses on cryoprecipitate.

When cryoprecipitate was analyzed, the following parameters besides
VIII:C and total protein were usually determined: Factor VIII-related
antigen (VIIIR:Ag) by immunoradiometric assay as described by Hellings
et al. (10); fibrinogen by a gravimetric method according to Strengers
and Asberg (11); fibronectin by radial immunodiffusion.

Controlled pore glass adsorption

The source material used for the studies with CPG consisted of small
amounts of cryoprecipitate obtained in bulk during routine production of
the present factor VIII concentrate. The standard conditions for assessing the optimum and acceptable range of every parameter under investigation were as follows:
— buffer: 20 mM Na$_3$-citrate, 60 mM NaCl, 3% (w/v) glucose, pH 6.8;
  two volumes of buffer per volume of cryo;
— CPG: 4 volumes of wet CPG (in buffer) per 3 volumes of cryosolution;
— adsorption: batchwise during 15 minutes at room temperature by
  turning a 10 ml tube end over end;
— washing/elution: columnwise, with starting buffer.
The starting cryoprecipitate solution and the CPG effluent were
analyzed for VIII:C and total protein.

CPG and chemicals

CPG was purchased from Sigma Chemical Co. (St. Louis, Mo.; CPG
500-200).
Chemicals were the highest purity grade available and purchased from
commercial sources.

RESULTS

Influence of freezing on factor VIII, salt and proteins

The experiments on the freezing of plasma showed that high concentrations of Na$^+$ and proteins were generated when the plasma was frozen
slowly. A typical example is shown in Figure 1, where a 2-fold increase
in concentrations is shown at the end of the freezing process for the
larger type of bag, with an even more pronounced effect for the smaller
bag. The molecular weight of the components however, did not appear
to have an influence on the extent of accumulation. The factor VIII

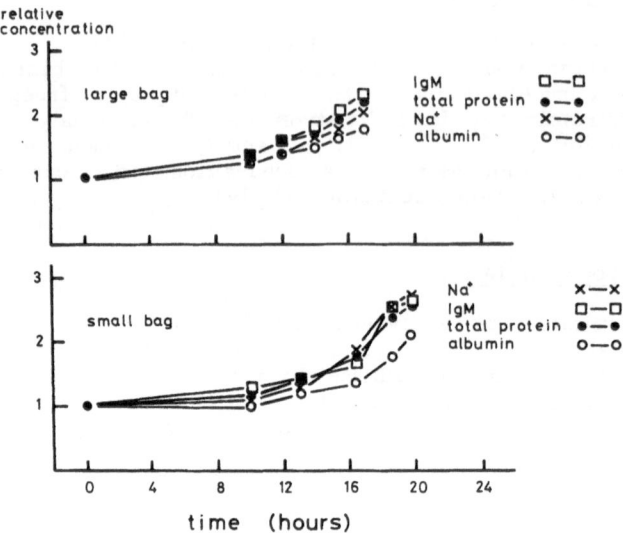

Figure 1. Accumulation of plasma constituents induced by freezing. The freezing regime consisted of laying two types of bags filled with 300 ml of plasma insulated in a polystyrene foam box in stationary air of -30°C. Samples of 1 ml were drawn from the centre of the bag at several timepoints during freezing.

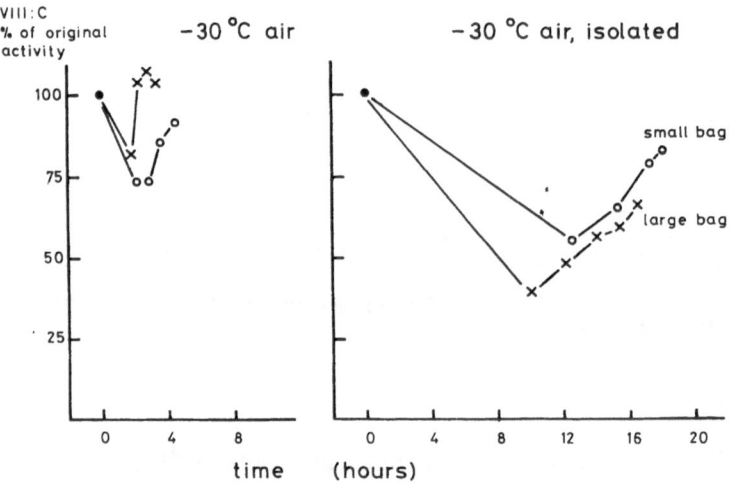

Figure 2. Behaviour of factor VIII in plasma during freezing. Freezing regimes consisted of laying two types of bags filled with 300 ml of plasma in stationary air of -30°C, or insulated in a polystyrene foam box in stationary air of -30°C. Samples of 1 ml were drawn from the centre of the bag at several timepoints during freezing.

complex showed a different behaviour however (fig. 2). In the course of freezing VIII:C decreased due to spontaneous cryoprecipitate formation and subsequent sedimentation, as assessed by measurements of VIIIR:Ag. At the end of the freezing process a rise to (near-) normal levels was observed due to the concentrating effect by slow freezing, but the specific activity remained low due to the high protein concentrations.

Table 1. Influence of freezing rate on VIII:C and protein recovery in cryoprecipitate

	recovery	VIII:C (IU/l)	protein mg/ml	fibrinogen mg/ml	spec.act. IU/mg
	cryo	sup.pl.			
− 30°C air, isolated	433*	140	34.9	14.6	0.21†
− 30°C stationary air	490	150	29.5	13.0	0.29±
− 100°C N_2 gas	513*	200	23.7	11.2	0.38
− 79°C CO_2/ethanol	467	190	23.2	10.5	0.34

Results are shown as the mean of 3 experiments in large bags and of 3 experiments in small bags. The mean VIII:C concentration in the starting plasma was 0.80 IU/ml.

* : recoveries being significantly different (P < 0.005, paired t test)
† : significantly different from 0.29 (P < 0.005) and 0.38 (P < 0.001)
± : significantly different from 0.38 (P < 0.005)

Table 1 shows the influence of the rate of freezing on the recovery and specific activity of VIII:C in cryoprecipitate. The effect on the recovery was not very pronounced, with only the lowest freezing rate yielding significantly lower figures than the freezing in CO_2-ethanol, but the specific activity was significantly lower for both low rates of freezing. Part of the increased amount of protein in the precipitate was caused by fibrinogen (table 1), but also fibronectin is expected to be an important factor (not measured).

As slow freezing generates salt gradients in the plasma and results in lower specific activities, the effect of extra salt addition to plasma prior to (rapid) freezing was investigated. It turned out that with increasing salt concentrations (up to 1 M added) VIII:C recoveries in cryo decreased, while more VIII:C was detected in the cryosupernatant. VIIIR:Ag measurements revealed that VIII:C dissociated from the VIIIR:Ag with increasing salt concentrations, while precipitation of total protein was promoted. Contrary to that, removal of salt from plasma by dialysis against distilled water (containing 10 mM citrate) caused a shift of VIII:C from the cryosupernatant to the cryoprecipitate leading to recoveries of VIII:C of 495 IU/l (n = 7) in the cryoprecipitate, which was significantly better than the 390 IU/l for the controls. The specific activity of VIII:C remained the same however, as also more protein was recovered in the cryoprecipitate of dialyzed plasma.

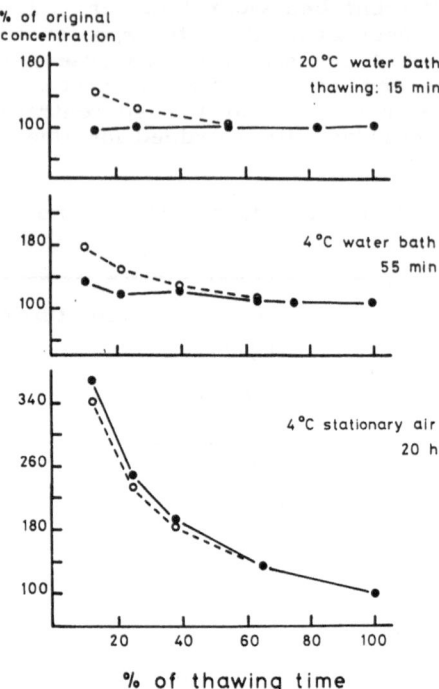

Figure 3. Concentrations of plasma constituents in the fluid phase of thawing plasma. The concentrations shown are the mean of the concentrations of Na⁺, albumin, IgG, IgA, IgM and total protein. The broken line represents the data for plasma that had been frozen slowly (4-6 hours), the solid line those for quickly frozen plasma (10 minutes).

Influence of thawing on factor VIII, salt and proteins

Plasma bags frozen in a fast and in a slow way were thawed in different media and the liquid phase formed was analyzed for salt and proteins. Using a quick thaw process the composition of the fluid phase from quickly frozen plasma was homogeneous all over the thawing time (fig. 3), while concentrations of salt and protein were higher than originally present, when the plasma had been frozen slowly. With longer thawing times however, this difference was not present, but initial concentrations then were much higher than the original ones. Similar findings were obtained in thaw-siphoning which implies that at the end of the thawing process the composition of the effluent was still the original one when the plasma had been frozen fast, but did hardly contain any salt or protein, in case the plasma had been frozen slowly (not shown). VIII:C concentrations in the thaw-siphon effluent were also higher in the first emerging fluid phase of slowly frozen plasma, pointing to a bigger loss of VIII:C in the cryoprecipitate compared to well-frozen plasma.

Table 2. Influence of thawing regime on recovery and specific activity of VIII:C.

Thawing condition + thawing time	Fast frozen plasma recovery VIII:C (IU/1)		Slowly frozen plasma recovery VIII:C (IU/1)		Spec. act IU/mg	
	cryo	sup.pl.	cryo	sup.pl.	fast	slow
Batchwise:						
20°C waterbath 15 min.	285	345	340	135	0.25	0.19
4°C waterbath 55 min.	385	200	350	135	0.24	0.15
4°C stationary air 20 h.	345	100	340	100	0.13	0.11
Thaw-siphon:						
7°C waterbath 27 min.	340	280	295	265	0.20	0.20
4°C waterbath 47 min.	415	230	300	220	0.25	0.18

Results are shown as the mean of 6 bags (cryo of 2 bags pooled in each of 3 experiments). The mean VIII:C concentration in the starting plasma was 0.70 IU/ml.

Table 2 shows the influence of the way and rate of thawing on the recovery and specific activity of factor VIII in cryoprecipitate. Optimal conditions for both batchwise thawing and thaw-siphoning consisted of a waterbath of 4°C. When the plasma had been frozen fast, VIII:C recoveries and specific activities were then maximal. Also, no difference existed then between the performance of batchwise thawing and thaw-siphoning.

In a subsequent study using waterbathes of different temperatures, a thawing condition of a 7°C waterbath for thaw-siphoning was optimal in terms of process time, VIII:C recovery and specific activity in cryo-precipitate. In routine practice, however, a 4-6°C rocking waterbath will be the condition of choice.

Preparation of high purity factor VIII concentrate by CPG

CPG has been applied in the preparation of a factor VIII concentrate from cryoprecipitate, yielding a preparation with a purity of about 1 IU/mg and a final recovery of about 240 IU/1 (3, 4). The recovery relative to cryoprecipitate in the adsorption step was reported to be in the range of 80-100% depending on the purity wanted. As our present production of factor VIII concentrate (with a specific activity of 1.3 IU/mg on average) has a recovery of 160 IU/1 only, the CPG technique can contribute to solve the problem of shortage in the supply of fresh-frozen plasma for factor VIII production. A detailed investigation was started to establish for the CPG step the optimal conditions as well as their range that can be tolerated in routine processing. As an additional step to the method published, a concentrating step had to be developed to enable injection of a high dosis of VIII:C in a small volume.

The following processing conditions were investigated: pore diameter of CPG, ratio of CPG to cryo, inonic strength, pH, citrate concentration, presence of sugar, temperature and exposure time. Of these parameters inonic strength (O-250 mM NaCl), sugar content (O-5% w/v) and temperature (10-40°C) did not affect the performance of CPG over the ranges indicated. A citrate concentration of 40mM resulted in a slight decrease of the recovery and specific activity of VIII:C, but up to 20 mM no such effect was observed.

More critical were the pore diameter (cf. ref. 3), pH and exposure time. Using CPG from Sigma a pore diameter of 500 Å was optimal. The optimal pH was 6.6 with an acceptable working range of 6.2 to 8.0. The recovery of VIII:C decreased gradually with increasing exposure time (fig. 4). About 30 minutes to 1 hour were needed for maximal protein

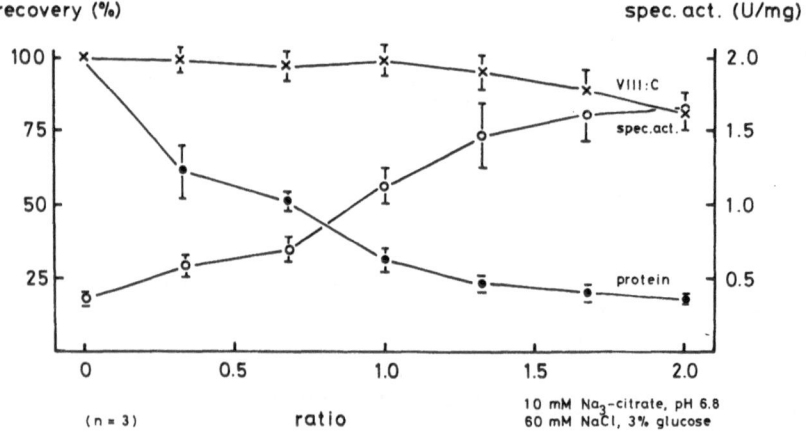

Figure 4. Adsorption patterns of VIII:C and total protein in cryoprecipitate as a function of varying ratio's of (wet) CPG over cryoprecipitate solution (1 volume of cryoprecipitate + 2 volumes of buffer). Mean and SD of 3 experiments are shown.

binding, but after 2 hours losses of VIII:C became significant. When exposure time was prolonged to 20 hours, only 20% was recovered, both of VIII:C and VIIIR:Ag, but total protein was unaffected. In routine practice exposure time was chosen to be 15 minutes, leaving more than one hour to complete the elution.

Not surprisingly, the ratio of CPG over cryo had a big impact on both the purity and recovery of VIII:C (fig. 5). In our aim of obtaining a specific activity of 1-1.5 IU/mg a ratio of 1.3 volumes of wet CPG was required per volume of cryosolution (one volume of bulk cryo + 2 volumes of buffer). In this approach 1 ml of wet CPG binds 22-30 mg of protein. At higher ratio's higher purities were obtained, but at the cost of recoveries.

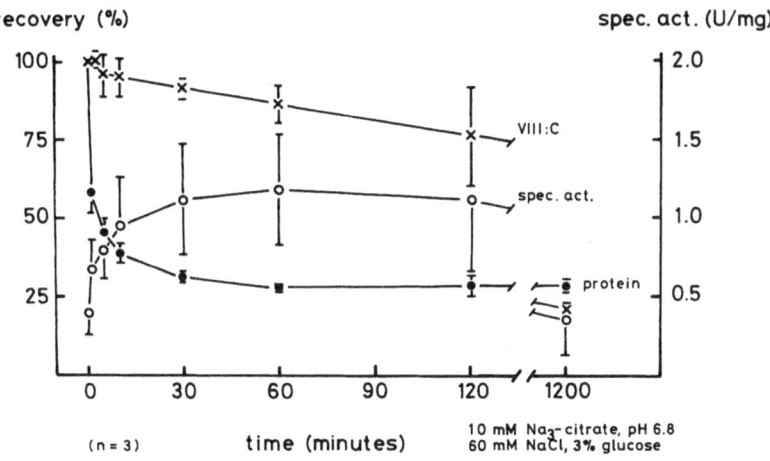

Figure 5. Adsorption patterns for VIII:C and total protein in cryoprecipitate as a function of exposure time. Mean and SD of
3 experiments are shown.

As concentrating techniques, to be applied on the CPG-effluent, ultrafiltration, glycine/NaCl-precipitation and polyethyleneglycol (PEG) precipitation were investigated. Of these possibilities ultrafiltration failed due to spontaneous protein precipitation induced by pumping the solution. Simultaneous addition of glycine and NaCl proved to be optimal at concentrations of 2 M and 2.5 M, respectively. VIII:C recoveries were about 90% in that step with the additional advantage of a 2-fold purification due to removal of immunoglobulins, albumin and some fibronectin. For obvious reasons desalting of the dissolved precipitate by gel filtration was required as an additional step.

Concentration by PEG-induced precipitation was another alternative. A final concentration of at least 7% (w/v) PEG-4000 at 0-4°C was sufficient to precipitate the factor VIII complex quantitatively (90% recovery), while total protein precipitated for only 50%. However, the final product formed a heavy precipitate after lyophilization and dissolution in water. This precipitate formation was eliminated to a large extent by including a precipitation at 4 or 5% (w/v) PEG-4000 at 20°C before

8% PEG was applied. The whole concentration procedure resulted in a recovery relative to cryoprecipitate of 65-70%, while the specific activity increased 3-fold to over 3 IU/mg (Table 3). After freeze-drying and dissolution protein did not precipitate heavily, but after 15-30 minutes protein threads were formed. Analysis of these threads revealed that fibrinogen and fibronectin were constituents, but other components cannot be excluded yet. Analysis of the protein composition at different stages of the fractionation procedure revealed that in the 5% PEG step mainly fibrinogen and IgM were removed. It should be noted that $Al(OH)_3$ adsorption does not seem to be necessary, but it can be combined with the 5% PEG step. Difficulties that are encountered up till now consist of significant losses of factor VIII during filtration and secondly, the protein instability after freeze drying and dissolution. Nevertheless, the reconstituted product shows excellent stability of factor VIII.

Table 3. Concentrating of CPG effluent in 2 PEG-steps

	recovery VIII:C (%)	spec.act. IU/mg
cryo	100	0.28 ± 0.05
CPG	100 ± 19	1.0 ± 0.2
5% PEG	81 ± 20	1.6 ± 0.8
8% PEG	67 ± 10	3.9 ± 0.6
filtered	53 ± 4	3.3 ± 0.9

Results are shown as the mean ± SD of 8 runs on laboratory scale. Recoveries are expressed relative to cryoprecipitate.

DISCUSSION

Three distinct, although related investigations have been described. The first one, dealing with the influence of freezing of plasma on factor VIII production, has shown that a fast freezing process is beneficial for the subsequent factor VIII fractionation. Although the impact on recovery is not dramatic, the specific activity of VIII:C in cryoprecipitate is strongly influenced by the rate of freezing. Cryoprecipitate from quickly frozen plasma (when optimally thawed) will therefore require less effort in further purification to a final product of high purity.

Slow freezing of plasma generated salt and protein gradients, as was also reported by Chang (12). Salt was found to negatively influence VIII:C recoveries in cryoprecipitate. Our conclusion therefore is, that although cryoprecipitation of fibrinogen, fibronectin and other proteins may be based on a salting-out effect (13), cryoprecipitation of VIII:C is not, but rather is a cold-induced, still poorly defined process. Although in the set-up of the study no freezing regimes were applied that yielded freezing times between 15 minutes and 3 hours, we feel that fresh plasma in bags should be frozen within 30 minutes, which corresponds to a freezing rate of at least 3 cm/hour.

The second study on the influence of the thawing rate revealed similar phenomena as in the previous one. A low thawing rate induced formation of salt and protein gradients and led also to low recoveries and specific activities of VIII:C. The influence on the recovery however, was more pronounced than in the case of freezing. It is therefore clear that for optimal factor VIII production both freezing and thawing should be fast processes. Limitations are set however, to the rate of thawing due to the necessity to keep the temperature of the thawed phase below 8°C. An optimal thawing condition in our hands consisted of a (rocking) waterbath of 4-6°C.

It was also found that when both freezing and thawing were fast processes, there was no significant difference in terms of factor VIII between batchwise thawing and thaw-siphoning. When the plasma had been frozen fast the protein and salt concentrations were equal to the original ones all over the thaw-siphoning time. So, no supervision was needed at the end of the thaw-siphon process to prevent a low osmolality in the final cryoprecipitate or loss of VIII:C as was observed earlier (6, 14). Our experience however was that thaw-siphoning, although attractive because no centrifugation is needed, is not practical on a large scale due to frequent clogging of the effluent tubing.

Finally, the CPG study has shown that substantial adsorption of the main contaminants in cryoprecipitate, fibrinogen and fibronectin, to glass surface can be carried out without significant loss of VIII:C.

The main losses of VIII:C in this approach occur at the level of cryoprecipitation and concentrating. The recoveries relative to cryoprecipitate are on average 50-60% which means that final recoveries are about 240 IU/l, as cryoprecipitation yield at present 450 IU/l plasma. However, some uncertainties for the future remain as the process up till now is run at a scale of only 10 liters of plasma. One may anticipate that losses in some steps will increase, while other, for instance in filtration, may become less pronounced.

The final preparation dissolves in about 2 minutes, is very stable on the bench, highly concentrated and has a relatively high specific activity. After dissolving, the solution is clear, but the problem that still remains to be solved is the apparent instability of some protein, most likely being fibrinogen and fibronectin. Present research is now ongoing to overcome this last difficulty after which the process can be scaled up and clinical evaluation be started.

REFERENCES

1. Report of a Working Party of the Regional Transfusion Directors Committee. Variables involved in cryoprecipitate production and their effect of factor VIII activity. Br J Haematol 1979;43:287-95.
2. Vermeer C. Soute BAM, Ates G, Brummelhuis HGJ. Contributions to the optimal use of human blood. VII. Increase of the yield of factor VIII in four-donor cryoprecipitate by an improved processing of blood and plasma. Vox Sang 1976;30:1-22.
3. Margolis J, Rhoades PH. Preparation of high-purity factor VIII by controlled pore glass chromotography. Lancet 1981;ii:446-9.
4. Margolis J, Gallovich CM, Rhoades P. A process for preparation of 'high-purity' factor VIII by controlled pore glass treatment. Vox Sang 1984;46:341-8.
5. Mason EC. Thaw-siphon technique for production of cryoprecipitate concentrate of factor VIII. Lancet 1978;ii:15-7.
6. Prowse CV, McGill A. Evaluation of the 'Mason' (continuous-thaw-siphon) method for cryoprecipitate production. Vox Sang 1979;37: 235-43.

7. Veltkamp JJ, Drion EF, Loeliger EA. Detection of the carrier state in hereditary coagulation disorders I. Thromb Diath Haemorrh 1968;19:279-303.
8. Over J. Methodology of the one-stage assay of factor VIII (VIII:C). Scand J Haematol 1984;33(Suppl.41):13-24.
9. Out TA, McDonald JR, Woldhuis-Kant J, Nieuwenhuys EJ. The effect of reduction of IgM on the quantitative determination of IgM by radial immunodiffusion and turbidimetry. Clin Chim Acta 1984; 144:115-26.
10. Hellings JA, Over J, van Mourik JA. The effect of storage of whole blood on the association of factor VIII-related antigen and factor VIII-coagulant antigen. Scand J Haematol 1982;29:353-62.
11. Strengers T, Asberg EGMT. Een screening-test, gevolgd door een snelle kwantitatieve microbepaling van fibrinogeen in plasma. Ned T Geneesk 1963;44:2044-5.
12. Chang CE. Segregation of proteins and sodium in human plasma upon freezing. Vox Sang 1983;44:238-45.
13. Polson A. Mechanism of cryoprecipitation. Prep Biochem. 1972;2:53-9.
14. Kang EP. An improved thaw-siphon method for the cryoprecipitate preparation. Vox Sang 1980;38:172-7.

CHROMATOGRAPHIC METHODS OF PLASMA FRACTIONATION

J.M. Curling

Plasma fractionation on a large scale (batch sizes 1000-5000 litres) is still carried out on the basis of the methods 6 and 9 developed by E.J. Cohn. However, cold ethanol precipitation is generally restricted to the production of albumin and intra-muscular IgG. Of all the other plasma proteins produced for therapeutic use, Factor VIII is probably the only protein not produced on a routine basis by chromatography. Thus factor IX concentrate, antithrombin III, fibronectin, C-1 esterase inhibitor are produced chromatographically as side fractions of ethanol precipitation (1). For these proteins and for specific immune globulins, especially anti-D(Rh) IgG, ion exchange or affinity chromatography are the current methods of choice.

When used in conjunction with ethanol fractionation chromatography is often used, initially, as a simple adsorption step causing as little delay as possible to the main (bulk) fractionation. Thus factor IX complex is adsorbed to DEAE-Sephadex A-50 and antitrombin III to Heparin-Sepharose. In each case conditions have been found that do not alter the ionic, protein or other chemical compositions of the plasma to be subject to ethanol precipitation. These are essentially batch adsorption methods but elution of the protein is often carried out from the 'cake' in a column or column-like procedure using simple buffer systems (2).

Although ion exchangers have been used for decentralized anti-D IgG production since the early 1970's (3) it was not until 1980 that large scale chromatographic fractionation for albumin came into routine use (4). Because of the mandatory pasteurization at 60°C for 10 h of all albumin preparations the possible presence of hepatitis infectivity was considered a limitation in the use of chromatography. Nor was it considered limiting for chromatographic preparation of anti-D IgG but for the reason that this protein was prepared from small pools from clearly identifiable female donors carefully monitored and known not to be HBsAg positive.

Albumin is generally prepared by methods based on sequential ion exchange chromatography first described in 1977 (5). Initial work was done on fractionation of up to 16 litre batches of plasma. Multiple cycles on 16 litre ion exchange columns allowed, by 1980, the fractionation of up to 250 litres of plasma per week (4). There are now several plants working in routine production of albumin for which clinical trial data is now available. These production units are in South Africa, Yugoslavia and Hungary. Scale-up work has been carried out since 1981 and it has now been demonstrated that 1000-1500 litres of plasma can be fractionated per week on 16 litre columns using high flow rate ion exchangers (6).

The method used at CRTS, Lille is a combination of chromatography and ethanol precipitation. After isolation of Factor VIII, Factor IX and Antithrombin III, fraction II + III is precipitated at 19% ethanol. Ethanol in the supernatant III is partially removed by ultrafiltration and then subject to chromatography on DEAE-Sepharose Fast Flow, CM-Sepharose Fast Flow. The CM-supernatant is concentrated from 3% to 10% protein and chromatographed on Sephacryl S-200 to remove polymers, pyrogens and vasoactive substances. Using guinea pig ileum and rat models it has been shown that vasoactive substances are absent: in addition the chromatographic albumin shows lower endotoxin levels than Cohn albumin in quantitative L.A.L. tests. About 300 kgs of chromatographic albumin have been injected into patients, especially in therapeutic plasma exchange where it shows improved tolerance over the ethanol fractionated material.

In addition the Skopje Transfusion Service has published the following data (7) on albumin produced entirely by chromatography. Albumin was given to 547 patients for the following indications: Shock (373), burns (7), liver cirrhosis (56), sepsis (6), malignancy (24), newborn with hyperbilirubinaemia (56), EPH-gestosis (25). Adverse reactions — hyperthermia, hypertension and tachycardia — were found in 11 patients but could not be related to pyrogen levels in the products. This insitute concludes that their product fulfills US, European and British Pharmacopoeia requirements and is well tolerated. The process yields a product of more than 99% purity and 80% recovery.

A totally chromatographic route for the integrated production of albumin and IgG has been developed by Friesen (8). DEAE and CM ion exchange cascades are used for both products. Final gel filtration of the albumin is not used. The Winnipeg plant, which is capable of fractionating 1600 litres/week in 800 litre batches, represents a significant advance in chromatographic fractionation. Friesen has reported (8) on at least 10^4 reduction of HBsAg activity to below the sensitivity of the Austria II method over the two anion exchange steps used. Similar data have also been reported comparing the capacities of QAE and DEAE derivatives of dextran, agarose and porous silica (9). QAE-Sephadex and DEAE-Sephadex showed higher affinity for HBsAg than DEAE-Sepharose and the DEAE-dextran derivative of Spherosil. This latter material, however, has shown high efficiency in the preparation of placental albumin of very high purity and clinical tolerance (10).

It is significant and to be expected that the chromatographic pathways to prepare IgG yield a product suitable for intravenous use. This has been demonstrated by Walsh et al. (11) and many others including Friesen (12). However, most of these products are hyperimmune globulins. More recently it has been shown that chromatography can be applied to the production of an intravenous, normal IgG (13). In this method reported by Berglöf, which can be totally integrated with the chromatographic purification of albumin (14), the IgG fraction for albumin production is rechromatographed in a two tandem-column procedure. The first column is a mixture 60/40 of DEAE-Sepharose Fast Flow and Arginine-Sepharose. The IgG is finally purified on CM-Sepharose Fast Flow. The method yields an intact, native monomeric IgG free of prekallikrein activator. Traces of plasmin and plasminogen may be detected. However, the product is highly stable on storage.

The large scale chromatographic methods referenced here clearly indicate that much progress has been made in the last four years (1980-1984) and that chromatography is applicable for albumin and IgG production on a routine basis up to at least 1500 litres/week and that these products show a clinical record of safety and tolerance.

REFERENCES

1. Brummelhuis HGJ. UNIDO Symposium, Stockholm 1982.
2. Wickerhauser M, Williams CG. A single-step method for the isolation of antithrombin III. Vox Sang. 1984;47:397-405.

3. Hoppe HH, Mester T, Hennes W, Krebs JJ. Prevention of Rh immunization: modified production of IgG anti-Rh for intravenous application by ion exchange chromatography. Vox Sang. 1973;25: 308-16.
4. Viljoen M, Shapiro M, Crookes R, Chalmers A, Marrs S. Large scale recovery of human serum albumin by a chromatographic method. Abstracts 17th Congress ISBT Budapest Akamdémiai Nyomda, 1982: 296.
5. Curling JM, Berglöf J. Lindquist LO, Eriksson S. A chromatographic procedure for the purification of human plasma albumin. Vox Sang. 1977;33:97-107.
6. Martinache L, Henon MP, Goudemand M. Large scale production of human albumin by chromatography, processed automatically. Abstracts 18th Congress ISBT. S. Karger, Basel 1984:156.
7. Damevska O, Ivanovski D, Dejanov I, Kolevski P. Preparation and use of human albumin produced by large scale chromatography. Abstracts 18th Congress ISBT. S. Karger, Basel 1984:158.
8. Friesen AD, Bowman JM, Bees WCH. Elution of HBsAg during ion exchange chromatographic production of albumin and immune serum globulin for intravenous use. Abstracts 18th Congress ISBT. S. Karger, Basel, 1984:161.
9. Zolton RP, Padvelskis JV. Evaluation of an anion-exchange procedure for removal of hepatitis type B contamination from human gamma globulin products. Vox Sang. 1984;47:114-21.
10. Eygonnet JP, Buffat JJ, Giroud M. et al. Clinical tolerance of human albumin. Abstracts 17th Congress ISBT Budapest. Akamdémiai Nyomda, 1982:316.
11. Walsh TJ, O'Riordan JP. A review of the production and clinical use of intravenous anti-D immunoglobulin. Ir. Med. J. 1982;75:243-4.
12. Friesen AD, Bowman JM, Price HW. Column ion exchange preparation and characterization of an Rh immune globulin (WIN Rho) for intravenous use. J. Appl. Biochem. 1981;3:164-75.
13. Berglöf JH, Eriksson S. Improvements in chromatographic preparation of human immunoglobulin G. Abstracts 18th Congress ISBT. S. Karger, Basel 1984:160.
14. Berglöf JH, Eriksson S, Curling JM. Chromatographic preparation and in vitro properties of albumin from human plasma. J. Appl. Biochem. 1983;5:282-92.

POLYELECTROLYTE FRACTIONATION TECHNOLOGY

S.M. Middleton

INTRODUCTION

A series of solid phase polyelectrolytes based on ethylene maleic anhydride co-polymer have been used to develop a flexible integrated system for the fractionation of plasma (1).

A high density polyelectrolyte designated PE 100 has been shown to be effective for the preparation of concentrates of albumin gammaglobulin and factors II, VII, IX and X. A low charge density polyelectrolyte designated PE 5 has been found to be a highly specific adsorbant for the factor VIII clotting moiety. PE 5 is being applied extensively to the production of novel high purity concentrates of factor VIII:C of both Human en Porcine origin. The application of this technology will be reviewed.

ETHYLENE MALEIC ANHYDRIDE (EMA) POLYELECTROLYTES

EMA polyelectrolytes are a series of reagents in which the anhydride groups have been substituted with a positively charged diethyl amino propylimide group (DMAPI). The degree of substitution can be varied to achieve a series of reagents with different charge densities.

Where 100% of the available anhydride groups are substituted with the positively charged group, the polyelectrolyte is designated PE 100. Where only 5% of the available anhydride groups are substituted with the DMAPI group the polyelectrolyte which consequently has a much lower charge density is designated PE 5. In this instance the remaining anhydride groups are 'blocked' with a non-reactive imide.

EMA polyelectrolytes can be used in either a column or batch mode. They are heat and acid stable and can consequently be re-cycled for re-use.

APPLICATION OF PE 100 TO THE FRACTIONATION OF PLASMA

EMA Polyelectrolytes PE 100 and PE 5 have been applied in an integrated system to the fractionation of Human plasma (fig. 1). The steps shown have the potential to be performed independently or in conjunction with another fractionation scheme.

Essentially PE 100 in common with other ion exchange resins will adsorb protein through electrostatic interaction between negatively charged protein and the positively charged resin; the protein can be subsequently eluted by adjustment of the pH or ionic strength to minimise the electrostatic charge on either protein or PE. For example, albumin is adsorbed from diluted plasma at pH 7.0 when the negative charge of the albumin is maximised. By lowering the pH to 4.0, which is below the isoelectric point of the albumin, the protein is readily eluted.

It is reported that albumin can be purified from plasma at a yield of 92% at 98.5% purity using this technology (1). By contrast gamma-globulin with a high isoelectric point (pl 7.5) will not bind to the polyelectrolyte; gammaglobulin can be concentrated from the PE Supernatant fraction at a yield of 92% at 97.5% purity (1). Factors II, VII, IX and X can be adsorbed directly from undiluted plasma to PE 100. These, like albumin, are relatively small proteins with an acid pH and consequently are readily adsorbed to the PE at pH 7.0. They can be eluted by increase in ionic strength.

PLASMA

| | E100 Adsorption
pH 7.8 | Elute
pH 6.0 | FII VII IX and X |

SUPERNATANT

| | E5 Adsorption
pH 6.5 | Elute
pH 6.7 | FVIII:C |

SUPERNATANT

| | E100 Adsorption
pH 6.0 | Elute
pH 6.0 | FVIIIR:COF
FVIIIR:Ag |

SUPERNATANT
  Dilute with H_2O

| | E100 Adsorption
pH 6.0 | Elute
pH 4.0 | Albumin |

SUPERNATANT
  Concentrate

GAMMA GLOBULIN

Figure 1. Fractionation of Plasma using EMA Polyelectrolytes

By contrast the high molecular weight factor VIII, although readily adsorbed to the PE 100, cannot be effectively eluted. It has been hypothesised that this is possibly due to the formation of multiple binding sites between the large protein and the polyelectrolyte.

APPLICATION OF PE 5 TO THE PURIFICATION OF FACTOR VIII

It has been shown that the factor VIII clotting moiety (FVIII:C) can be adsorbed to and effectively eluted from the low charge density poly-electrolyte PE 5. The factor VIII related antigen (factor VIII R:Ag) is retained in the PE 5 Supernatant.
  This fractionation of moieties of the factor VIII complex results in the production of a novel concentrate that is enriched in factor VIII:C and relatively depleted in factor VIII R:Ag.

FRACTIONATION OF HUMAN CRYOPRECIPITATE USING PE 5

Attempts have been made to purify factor VIII:C directly from plasma using PE 5. It has been observed that even with prior removal of the vitamin K dependent clotting factors using $AL(OH)_3$ or PE 100, factor VIII:C prepared directly from plasma displays inherent instability.

The fractionation of cryoprecipitate using PE 5 has been extensively studied.

Cryoprecipitate is dissolved in isontonic Tris buffered saline pH 7.0 and adsorbed with $Al(OH)_3$ prior to application to the Polyelectrolyte.

The cryoprecipitate is applied to the PE resin which is contained in a short column. After adsorption of the factor VIII:C the supernatant protein is removed by extensive washing. The factor VIII clotting activity is eluted using 1M NaCl, and subsequently concentrated from the eluate by precipitation with polyethylene glycol or by ultrafiltration. It has been observed that the use of sodium chloride at a concentration in excess of 1.0M inhibits elution of factor VIII:C indicating that the adsorption of factor VIII:C to PE 5 is possibly due to a combination of hydrophobic and ionic interactions. The results of the fractionation of cryoprecipitate are shown in Table 1. The specificity of the PE 5 for the factor VIII:C is clearly illustrated by the very low recovery of protein and in particular factor VIII R:Ag in the column eluate.

A profile of the PE purified factor VIII:C compared to the cryoprecipitate source is shown in Table 2. As can be seen a 40 fold purification of factor VIII:C relative to total protein is achieved over processing. Specifically levels of fibrinogen, IgG and IgM are reduced. As indicated earlier IgG and IgM will not bind to the positively charged polyelectrolyte and consequently a reduction in the concentration of these proteins, in which the blood group isoagglutinins are identified, would be expected over processing.

Table 1. Fractionation of human cryoprecipitate using EMA polyelectrolyte PE5

| N = 7 | % Recovery from Cryoprecipitate | | |
	Total Protein	Factor VIII:C	Factor VIII R:Ag
PE E5			
Supernatant	84.3 ± 6.8	21.7 ± 8.6	64.7 ± 18
PE Eluate	1.01 ± 0.18	37.4 ± 5.7	1.27 ± 0.8

FRACTIONATION OF HEPATITIS B SURFACE ANTIGEN AND HBV USING POLYELECTORLYTE PE 5

Cryoprecipitate has been deliberately contaminated with serum containing Hepatitis B Surface Antigen and HBV-DNA. The fractionation of these entities on PE 5 has been studied (2). I^{125} labelled HBsAg was added to cryoprecipitate and the cryoprecipitate fractionated on the PE 5 using standard methodology. The I^{125} label was monitored in the supernatant, wash and eluate fractions from the column. It was observed that the I^{125} label was detectable in the supernatant and wash fractions only, indicating that HBsAg was not binding to the PE 5. To ensure the integrity of the HBsAG I^{125} label, the peak fractions were incubated with a murine monoclonal antibody to HBsAg. Subsequently immune complexes were precipitated with a goat anti-mouse antibody. Using this technique 98.7% of the I^{125} activity was precipitated indicating that the I^{125} label was still bound to the HBsAg.

Table 2. Profile of polyelectrolyte purified human factor VIII:C

	Source cryoprecipitate	Polyelectrolyte fractionated human FVIII:C
Factor VIII:C (units/ml)	2.3	59.0
Factor VIII R:Ag (units/ml)	12.0	3.8
Protein (mg/ml)	9.0	7.2
Purity (units FVIII:C/mg protein)	0.23	8.2
Fibrinogen (mg/ml)	4.0	1.4
IgM (mg/ml)	0.24	<0.14
IgG (mg/ml)	0.6	<0.125
Isoagglutinins A_1	1/2	1/4
Isoagglutinins B	1/2	1/4
Solubility	Not measured	130 seconds

HBV-DNA was added to cryoprecipitate and using a molecular hybridisation assay, it was found that HBV-DNA is similarly excluded from the polyelectrolyte and could be recovered in the column supernatant but not in the column eluate.

These results indicated that the levels of HBsAg and HBV-DNA in cryoprecipitate could be reduced by fractionation over PE 5. However, only by extensive clinical trial can these observations be validated.

PHARMACOKINETICS OF POLYELECTROLYTE DERIVED HUMAN FACTOR VIII:C

A batch of polyelectrolyte derived Human Factor VIII:C has been prepared in order to establish pharmacokinetics and clinical efficacy.

Three patients with Hemophilia A and one with Von Willebrands disease were infused on separate occasions with Human PE VIII and conventional Intermediate Purity Factor VIII. The data which has been reported in detail by Tuddenham et al (3) indicate that the two types of FVIII concentrate have comparable pharmacokinetics and efficacy in patients with Hemophilia A. However, in the patient with Von Willebrands disease a half life of only 2½ hours was observed when Human PE VIII was infused. These results suggest that in vivo the presence of factor VIII R:Ag is necessary as a carrier for factor VIII:C.

In two patients with Hemophilia A, hemarthroses were treated with Human PE VIII, in both patients resolution was comparable to that which would be anticipated using a conventional concentrate of FVIII.

PURIFICATION AND CHARACTERISATION OF HUMAN FACTOR VIII:C

Human PE VIII has provided a unique source of enriched factor VIII:C which has proved important as the starting fraction for a purification procedure which has resulted in the isolation of pure factor VIII:C protein with a molecular weight of 365K (4).

In a collaborative project with Genentech Inc. in the U.S.A. this protein has been used to elucidate the primary structure of FVIII:C. Subsequently it has been possible to construct the gene for this very large protein with the result that authentic FVIII:C has now been synsthesised in mammalian cell culture.

FRACTIONATION OF PORCINE CRYOPRECIPITATE USING PE 5

Therapeutic concentrates of animal derived factor VIII have been available since the mid 1950's when they were used in the management of bleeding in hemophiliacs undergoing major surgery (5). More recently they have been used in patients who have developed an inhibitor to Human factor VIII:C. However, several problems were associated with the therapeutic use of these early concentrates. The low purity of the product resulted in poor solubility and a tendency to cause severe transfusion reactions with progressive 'resistance' after 6 days of therapy. Additonally the infusion of porcine and bovine derived products could provoke serious thrombocytopenia. This was believed to be related to the presence in the product of factor VIII related platelet aggregating factor (FVIIIP:AgF), the functional activity associated with Porcine factor VIII R:Ag. It has been shown that FVIIIP:AgF will aggregate human platelets in the absence of risctocetin (6).

PE 5 is being used commercially to fractionate Porcine cryoprecipitate. The polyelectrolyte is being used in a routine large scale procedure in which cryoprecipitate containing 500,000 units of factor VIII:C is applied to 4 Kg of polyelectrolyte. The fractionation of Porcine cryoprecipitate using PE 5 is shown in Table 3. As can be seen, polyelectrolyte fractionation significantly reduces the levels of contaminating protein; the purity of the factor VIII:C has been increased 167 fold over the source cryoprecipitate. In addition the levels of factor VIII R:Ag and consequently factor VIII P:AgF are significantly reduced over processing.

This product has been used clinically over the last four years for the treatment of patients with an inhibitor to Human factor VIII:C. Clinical efficacy in these patients has been clearly established. There has been a significant reduction in the incidence of the transfusion reactions and 'resistance' phenomena that were associated with earlier concentrates of Porcine FVIII and the incidence of thrombocytopenia is negligible (7)(8).

SUMMARY

Solid phase ethylene maleic anhydride polyelectrolytes have been evaluated on both experimental and manufacturing scale. Specifically the low charge density polyelectrolyte has been used in the preparation of novel concentrates of factor VIII:C. Applied to the fractionation of Human cryoprecipitate the use of PE 5 has been found to result in reduced levels of contamination with total protein specifically fibrinogen and the blood group isoagglutinins and also agents relating to infectivity with Hepatitis B. Clinical efficacy has been demonstrated in a small number of patients.

PE is applied to the fractionation of Porcine cryoprecipitate in a routine manufacturing procedure and the final product is proving efficacious in the treatment of patients with inhibitors to Human factor VIII:C.

Table 3 Fractionation of Porcine Cryoprecipitate using EMA Polyelectrolyte PE 5

	Source cryoprecipitate	PE derived procine FVIII:C
Factor VIII:C (units/ml)	10.1	80.5
Factor VIIR:Ag (units/ml)	4.1	5.3
Factor VIIIP:AgF (units/ml)	2.0	1.6
Protein mg/ml	33	1.6
Specific activity (units FVIII:C/mg Protein)	0.3	50.3

REFERENCES

1. Johnson AJ, MacDonald VE, Semar M, et al. Preparation of the major plasma fractions by solid phase polyelectrolytes. J Lab Clin Med. 1976;922:194-210.
2. Galpin SA, Karayiannis P, Middleton SM, Thomas HC, The removal of Hepatitis B Virus from factor VIII concentrates by fractionation on Ethylene Maleic Anhydride Polyelectrolyte J. of Med. Virol. In Press.
3. Tuddenham EGD, Lane RS, Rotblat F et al. Response to infusions of polyelectrolyte fractionated human factor VIII concentrate in human Haemophilia A and Von Willebrands disease. Brit J Haemat 1982;52:259-67.
4. Rotblat F, O'Brien DP, Middleton SM, Tuddenham EGD. Purification and characterisation of human factor VIII:C. Thromb. Haemost. 1983;50:108.
5. Macfarlane RG, Mallam PC, Wills LJ et al. Surgery in haemophilia — The use of animal antihaemophilic globulin and human plasma in thirteen cases. Lancet 1957;ii:251.
6. Forbes CD, Prentice CMR. Aggregation of human platelets by purified porcine and bovine antihaemophilic factor. Nature New Biol. 1973;241:149.
7. Kernoff PBA, Thomas ND, Lilley PA et al. Clinical experience with polyelectrolyte fractionated porcine factor VIII concentrate in the treatment of Haemophiliacs with antibodies to factor VIII. Blood 1984;63:31-41.
8. Gatti L, Mannucci P. Use of porcine factor VIII in the management of seventeen patients with factor VIII antibodies. Thromb. Haemost. 1984;51:379-84.

RECOMBINANT DNA TECHNOLOGY FOR THE PRODUCTION OF PLASMA PROTEINS

W.D. Lake, W.R. Srigley

INTRODUCTION

During the past few years we have seen an unparalleled interest and growth in applied biology. The rapid progress in this area has been largely driven by laboratory advances in monoclonal antibody and recombinant DNA (r-DNA) techniques. Most of the early efforts to apply r-DNA technology to commercial product development were directed toward the production of small peptide hormones such as interferon, insulin and growth hormone. The only r-DNA produced therapeutic agent currently on the market is the human insulin preparation sold by Eli Lilly and Company. However, many observers believe that a human growth hormone preparation produced by Genentech could be available in 1985 and a number of other therapeutic agents such as tissue plasminogen activator are presently undergoing clinical trials.

Several biotechnology companies have announced independent or joint venture programs with established pharmaceutical companies to develop therapeutic plasma protein products using r-DNA techniques. In some cases these proteins are currently produced through the fractionation of human plasma. Other products under development represent new therapeutic agents for which no licensed production method exists. Although programs to produce human plasma derivates are still in the early stages, it is possible to speculate concerning the prospective impact of r-DNA technology on the production of plasma proteins; including which derivatives are likely to be replaced, what is the time prospect regarding the development of r-DNA plasma protein products and what are the clinical and regulatory aspects of bringing these products to market. For the most part, the present article will be confined to a consideration of the likely impact of r-DNA technology on the plasma protein market in the United States.

Two plasma derivatives frequently mentioned as targets for production using r-DNA techniques are Normal Serum Albumin (Human) and Antihemophilic Factor (Human), Factor VIII. These two products, along with Factor IX Complex (Human) and the various Immune Serum Globulin preparations, account for most of the present U.S.A. market in therapeutic plasma fractionation products. The estimated U.S.A. market size for these products is indicated in Table 1. Intravenous Gamma globulin has only recently been introduced in the United States. While the U.S.A. market for the product has not yet been developed, the combined IVIg market in West Germany and Japan is estimated to be 200 million U.S. dollars per year. This, along with the emerging interest in passive immunization as an acute and prophylactic therapy, leads one to anticipate that the potential sales in the U.S.A. for normal and hyper-immune globulins will grow substantially in the next few years. Considering the size of these already established markets it is not difficult to understand why biotechnology companies have selected plasma protein derivatives as target products to be developed through the new r-DNA technology.

Table 1. Estimated U.S.A. market for plasma derivatives*

Plasma derivative	Est. 1984 sales*
Serum Albumin	174
Antihemophilic (Human), Factor VIII	46
Factor IX Complex (Human)	13
Anti-Inhibitor Coagulant Complex (Activated factor IX)	11
Immune Serum Globulin	10
Intravenous Gamma Globulin	2

* In millions of U.S. Dollars.

HUMAN ALBUMIN

Based upon market size and the relative simplicity of the molecule, human serum albumin with a U.S.A. market of 174 million dollars is a particularly attractive product for recombinant technology. This protein is composed of 585 amino acid residues and has a molecular weight of approximately 66,000 (1). A molecule of this size no longer represents a difficult technical problem for an r-DNA approach. The fact that albumin is not a glycoprotein further simplifies the development of an r-DNA product identical to the native protein. In fact, human serum albumin has been cloned and expressed using r-DNA techniques by at least three biotechnology companies. At this time however, low expression levels coupled with difficulties in getting an organism to secrete albumin are yet to be overcome.

An approved Product License Application would be required to market an r-DNA produced human albumin in the United States. The Food and Drug Administration has indicated that all biotechnology derived products will be considered "New Drugs", even if the product is identical in molecular or chemical structure to a previously approved product produced by conventional methods (2). Thus, new license applications have been required for r-DNA derived insulin and growth hormone even though conventionally produced versions of these products are already marketed.

The amount of data required to support an application for an r-DNA produced product depends upon: (a) the proposed use of the product; (b) the degree to which the product resembles a previously approved product; (c) whether the administration of the product to patients would be episodal and infrequent or chronic; (d) the previous clinical experience with the conventionally produced product; and (e) the methods and materials used to prepare and purify the product. Based upon these criteria the clinical testing of an r-DNA derived human albumin identical to the conventionally produced product should not be an unusually lengthy or difficult process. Nevertheless these trials would probably require one and a half years in the U.S.A., and FDA review and approval of the Product License Application could easily require an additional year.

The key factor determining the time frame in which r-DNA technology will impact on the production of albumin may not be the clinical testing or regulatory aspects of bringing this product to market. It may instead be the development of process technology which allows r-DNA produced albumin to compete economically with large scale plasma fractionation.

Very large amounts of human albumin are produced in the U.S.A. through plasma fractionation. The 1984 requirement for human albumin in the United States was approximately six million units, which represents nearly 75,000 kilograms of protein. Albumin produced through an r-DNA process is not a new therapeutic agent and offers no obvious therapeutic advantage over the plasma derived product. This being the case, in order for the r-DNA product to make a significant impact on the albumin market either an increase in the market demand for albumin has to occur which cannot be satisfied by existing fractionation capacity, or the r-DNA process must result in a lower cost product than that produced through plasma fractionation. In the absence of any new or increased therapeutic applications of the product, significant expansion in market demand seems unlikely during the next five year period. Thus economics will probably be the factor which sets the pace for the application of the new technology.

To a great degree the cost of manufacturing plasma derivatives is determined by the cost and availability of plasma. One of the major advantages which r-DNA technology is expected to have over plasma fractionation is the possibility of producing products more economically using large scale fermentation methodology with raw materials less costly than plasma. The use of large scale fermentation processing would certainly be an essential requirement of a program to produce human albumin using biotechnology. In the near term however, competing with the economics of plasma fractionation may not be an easy task. Existing fractionation plants are quite efficient and experienced in the manufacture of plasma proteins. Even so, margins are not that great and in many markets albumin is sold as a commodity item.

In order to make a significant impact on the albumin plasma fractionation market a manufacturer producing albumin by an r-DNA process would probably have to have a production capacity of at least twenty percent of the total albumin market requirement. For the U.S.A. market this would mean a plant with an annual capacity of 15,000 kilograms of albumin. Using this target one can make some additional assumptions and calculate the required fermentation capacity of a manufacturing plant which could meet this demand. A reasonable cell density for a bacterial fermentation is about 5% wet weight and the total cell protein may be 50% of the wet cell mass (3). Assuming a cellular expression for albumin of 15% of total cell protein and a purification yield of 40% in the manufacturing process, then an r-DNA plant capable of producing 15,000 kilograms of albumin per year would have to have a fermentation capacity of approximately 100,000 liters. This plant would operate 330 days/yr. on a 3 day operating cycle. Depending upon location and other factors a capital investment of from $40-70 million U.S. dollars would be required to design and build such a plant and the construction time would require about three years. Staffing, training, validating and licensing the plant couls easily take one more year. This represents a very significant up front capital investement for the production by an alternate process of a product which is already sold as a commodity item. Of course, ignoring possible technical and regulatory barriers, the potential of leveraging excess fermentation capacity which may already exist could offer an alternative approach. The fact remains however that the r-DNA process must be price competitive with plasma fractionation to be successful and this is unlikely to be the case for some time. Thus, biotechnology will probably not play a significant role in the commercial production of human albumin much before 1995.

FACTOR VIII

The potential impact of r-DNA technology on the production of factor VIII on the other hand is very different from that for albumin. Factor VIII circulates in plasma as a complex glycoprotein with a molecular weight greater than one million (4). The factor VIII complex shows two distinct antigens; the factor VIII related antigen and the factor VIII clotting antigen. There are also two different biological activities; the factor VIII clotting activity and the factor VIII related ristocetin co-factor activity (5). The latter is reduced or absent in classical von Willebrand's disease while the factor VIII clotting activity is the biological activity lacking in hemophilia A. While the basic structure of the factor VIII complex and the exact relationship of the biological activities is still unknown, estimates of the molecular weight of the procoagulant protein, factor VIII:C, are in the 200,000 to 300,000 range (6). The clotting protein is present in plasma in only trace amounts which may be as low as 50 ng/ml. In commercial concentrates of factor VIII the clotting protein accounts for no more than 0.1 to 0.2% of the total protein of the concentrate and is thought to be stabilized by its binding to the factor VIIIR:Ag. The ratio of VIIIR:Ag to VIII:C activity in these products is around three to one (5).

The primary advantage of a recombinant DNA produced AHF would be the absence of risk of viral hepatitis or acquired immune deficiency syndrome (AIDS) now associated with the plasma derived concentrates. It is also possible that the r-DNA product might be less immunogenic than current therapeutic preparations. Approximately ten percent of hemophiliacs develop antibodies against factor VIII during the first year of treatment with the current preparations. The development of anti-factor VIII antibodies makes treatment more difficult and more expensive and can also be life threatening (7). Clearly however, the chronic life-long use of factor VIII requires that the known and manageable risks of the plasma derived product be the benchmark for evaluating the new generation products.

Preclinical and clinical testing of an r-DNA derived factor VIII will probably be more involved and will take longer than the testing of an r-DNA produced albumin. For a number of reasons r-DNA produced factor VIII is unlikely to be viewed as being identical to the conventionally produced plasma derived concentrate. The technical aspects of cloning and expressing the factor VIII procoagulant protein are also more challenging than with human albumin. Two biotechnology companies have reported the cloning and expression of factor VIII in the laboratory but the level of expression must be further increased to be commercially useful. Issues related to the purification process and the stability of the final drug product in the absence of the factor VIIIR:Ag must also be addressed. Furthermore, since AHF is administered repeatedly and perhaps prophylactically over many years there will be questions concerning potential long term effects associated with the use of the drug.

An advantage for the r-DNA approach to AHF manufacture in contrast to the use of the technology for albumin production is that a relatively small capital investment will be required for commercial manufacturing of an r-DNA factor VIII because of the low therapeutic dose required. Enough purified bulk factor VIII to supply the annual U.S.A. requirement could probably be produced in the space occupied by a single large laboratory room.

Assuming timely progress toward solving the remaining technical issues, clinical trials with an r-DNA produced factor VIII will probably begin in late 1985 or early 1986. If no difficult pharmacologic or safety issues arise, the r-DNA produced factor VIII could be licensed by 1990.

The U.S.A. market for factor VIII is estimated to be fifty million dollars per year and the world wide market is at least one hundred million dollars. This represents a very attractive potential market for a new drug. A therapeutically useful r-DNA produced, purified factor VIII could rapidly take market share from the established plasma derived concentrates and emerge as the drug of choice for the treatment of hemophilia A as early as 1992.

FACTOR IX

The market for plasma derived coagulation factor IX is smaller than that for factor VIII and the technical issues associated with producing this product using r-DNA methods are more complex. Factor IX has a molecular weight of approximately 56,000 with a carbohydrate content of 23%. One third of the carbohydrate is sialic acid (8). It is unlikely that an unglycosylated factor IX will have the same biological activity in vivo as the natural protein. Thus the r-DNA production of factor IX may depend upon the development of commercially useful mammalian cell lines which can secrete r-DNA proteins in the proper glycosylated form. Factor IX also contains γ-carboxylated glumatic acid residues which are introduced into the finished peptide chain in a vitamin K dependent reaction. These γ-carboxylated glumatic acid groups are essential for the biological activity of the protein (8). Present commercial factor IX concentrates derived from plasma also contain coagulation factors II, VII and X in addition to factor IX. The presence of small amounts of one or more of these additional factors may be important for the therapeutic activity of the factor IX concentrate. These factors makes the task of developing an economic large-scale manufacturing method even more challenging.

The clinical testing and regulatory aspects of bringing an r-DNA produced factor IX to market in the U.S.A. should be similar to those for factor VIII but the complexity of the factor IX molecule alone is enough to insure that its production by r-DNA technology will lag behind factor VIII. The production of factor IX by r-DNA technology could follow factor VIII by two to three years if the factor VIII product is commercially successful and if some difficult technical problems such as the γ-carboxylation of the molecule can be solved.

NEXT GENERATION

The plasma proteins considered above are the most likely first targets for commercial production using r-DNA methods. These products will probably not be available until the early 1990's. It is more difficult to predict the development time and likely success of other plasma protein products which may be produced by r-DNA methods.

It has been suggested that specific purified human immunoglobulins could be commercially produced using r-DNA methods. Researchers at Genentech have demonstrated the possibility of this approach by cloning and expressing the heavy and light chains of a monoclonal antibody molecule and then using these proteins to construct a functional anti-body in the laboratory (9). There are many technical problems which remain to be solved but the potential therapeutic value of large quantities of low cost human antibodies or combinations of antibodies for passive immunization and for treatment of specific diseases or infections is very significant.

Antithrombin III (AT III) is another plasma protein with therapeutic potential which could be produced by the r-DNA process in the future. Human Antithrombin III is a naturally occuring anticoagulant that specifically inhibits activated coagulation factors such as VIIa, IXa, Xa and XIIa (10). It may be of clinical value in treating disseminated intravascular coagulation (DIC), conditions where AT III is being rapidly consumed such as in acute or chronic liver disease or congenital deficiencies. Antithrombin III is a glycoprotein with a molecular weight of 55,000. The amino acid sequence is known (10). Baboon AT III has been cloned and could be used as a probe to isolate the corresponding human gene (10).

Programs to produce specific human immunoglobulins and Antithrombin III are still in very early stages. Market introduction of these plasma proteins produced through r-DNA technology will in all likelihood not occur before 1995.

CONCLUSION

Based upon the considerations outlined above, the commercial production of therapeutic plasma protein products using r-DNA methods is a technology of the 1990's. The first and most significant impact of recombinant DNA technology will probably be on factor VIII production while the timing for human albumin production will be determined by albumin market demand and r-DNA process economics. In fact, given the inter-relationship of the costs associated with the manufacture of products from plasma, it may be the market development of an r-DNA factor VIII product which makes r-DNA albumin commercially competitive with plasma derived product. If the demand for plasma based factor VIII were to decrease significantly, the cost of plasma now absorbed by factor VIII would be transferred to the remaining fractions, particularly albumin. It is also possible that the amount of albumin produced might decrease. Under these conditions, the price of plasma-derived albumin would likely rise. This would favorably impact the economics of investing in a large scale fermentation plant for albumin. Other plasma protein products such as factor IX, specific immunoglobulins and Antithrombin III are in the earliest stages of development using r-DNA methods. The many technical problems remaining to be solved lead one to conclude that these plasma proteins are unlikely to be commercially produced by r-DNA processing before 1995.

REFERENCES

1. Andersson L-O, Serum albumin, In: Blombäck B; Hanson LA, eds. Plasma Proteins. New York. John Wiley & Sons, 1979:43-71.
2. Food and Drug Administration. FDA talk paper T83-2: Regulating recombinant DNA products, January 7, 1983, Rockville, MD,: U.S. Department of Health and Human Services Public Health Service.
3. Bui PT. Recovery and purification of biologically active polypeptides from r-DNA microorganisms. Bio/Technology 1983;Aug:488-90.
4. Thomas KB, Howards MA, Koutts J. Firkin BG. Simplified Immunoradiometric assay for factor VIII coagulant antigen. Brit J Haemat 1982;51:47-57.
5. Barrowcliffe TW, Kemball-Cook G, Morris G, Holt JC, Furlong RA, Peake IR. Factor VIII related activities in therapeutic concentrates. J Lab Clin Med 1981;97:429-38.

6. Fulcher CA, Zimmerman TS. Characterization of the human factor VIII procoagulant protein with a heterologous precipitating antibody. Proc Natl Acad Sci USA 1982;1648-52.
7. Shapiro SS, Hultin M. Acquired inhibitors to the blood coagulation factors. Semin Thrombos Hemostas 1975;1:336-44.
8. Andersson L-O. Haemophilia B-factor (factor IX), In: Blombäck B, Hanson LA, eds. Plasma Proteins, New York. John Wiley & Sons, 1979:281-5.
9. Chase M. Genentech claims 'First' in technology to make anti-bodies: Firm, City of Hope medical scientists use techniques of Genetic engineering. Wall Street Journal 1983;May 5.
10. Stackhouse R, Chandra T, Robson KJH, Woo SLC. Purification of antithrombin III mRNA and cloning of its cDNA. J Biol Chem 1983;258:703-5.

COLUMN ION EXCHANGE CHROMATOGRAPHIC PRODUCTION OF ALBUMIN, IV ISG AND FACTOR IX FROM 75,000 TO 100,000 LITRES OF PLASMA PER YEAR

A.D. Friesen

INTRODUCTION

The Winnipeg Rh Institute is a private, non-profit institute incorporated in 1969. It's aims and objectives are to encourage and carry out research and development in de broadest sense, with particular interest in blood and blood products.

The Institute initially became involved in plasma fractionation in 1971 with the development of a column ion exchange chromatographic procedure for the production of Rh immune globulin (trade-named WinRho) for intravenous use using the DEAE Sephadex technique originally developed by Hoppe (1) of Hamburg, Germany. The process developed at the Winnipeg Rh Institute (2) is simple, recovering the Rh antibody from plasma at 91% efficiency, yields an immunoelectrophoretically pure IgG with less than 1% content of aggregated molecules, low anticomplement activity and low levels of IgA.

The success of this process encourages us to explore the use of ion exchange chromatography for the production of other hyper-immune globulins, as well as normal immune globulins, all for intravenous use. It was obvious, however, that the cost of discarding the DEAE Sephadex following each chromatographic run would be prohibitive for the production of normal immune serum globulin for intravenous (iv ISG) use. Consequently, we explored the use of more rigid ion exchange gels with the simultaneous production of albumin. Pilot scale studies were initiated in 1976 using 15 litre sectional columns with various ion exchange media including Sepharose, Biogel, Trisacryl, Fractogel and most recently Hema supports. The pilot scale studies resulted in the development of a chromatographic process for the production of iv ISG and albumin previously published (3-5). This ion exchange process has been integrated into a total fractionation process (fig. 1) which includes the production of intermediate purity factor VIII, factor IX, albumin and iv ISG at a scale of 800 litres per batch with the ability to process two or three batches per week. Construction of the Plasma Fractionation facility was completed in 1983 and is presently being commissioned with the clinical trials of all products scheduled to begin January 1985.

INDUSTRIAL SCALE PROCESS

The industrial scale process utilizes sanitary stationary stainless steel tanks connected with stainless steel piping, valves, pumps and sensors, all welded-in-place (fig. 2). The entire process is designed to be cleaned-in-place (CIP) with both the process and CIP systems fully automated. The stainless steel process is sited in a class 10,000 clean room and all tanks involved in the processing of plasma proteins are jacketted to provide maintenance of the protein solutions at 4-6°C. The process is designed and constructed to comply with the current Good Manufacturing Practices (GMP) regulations of the United States Food and Drug Association.

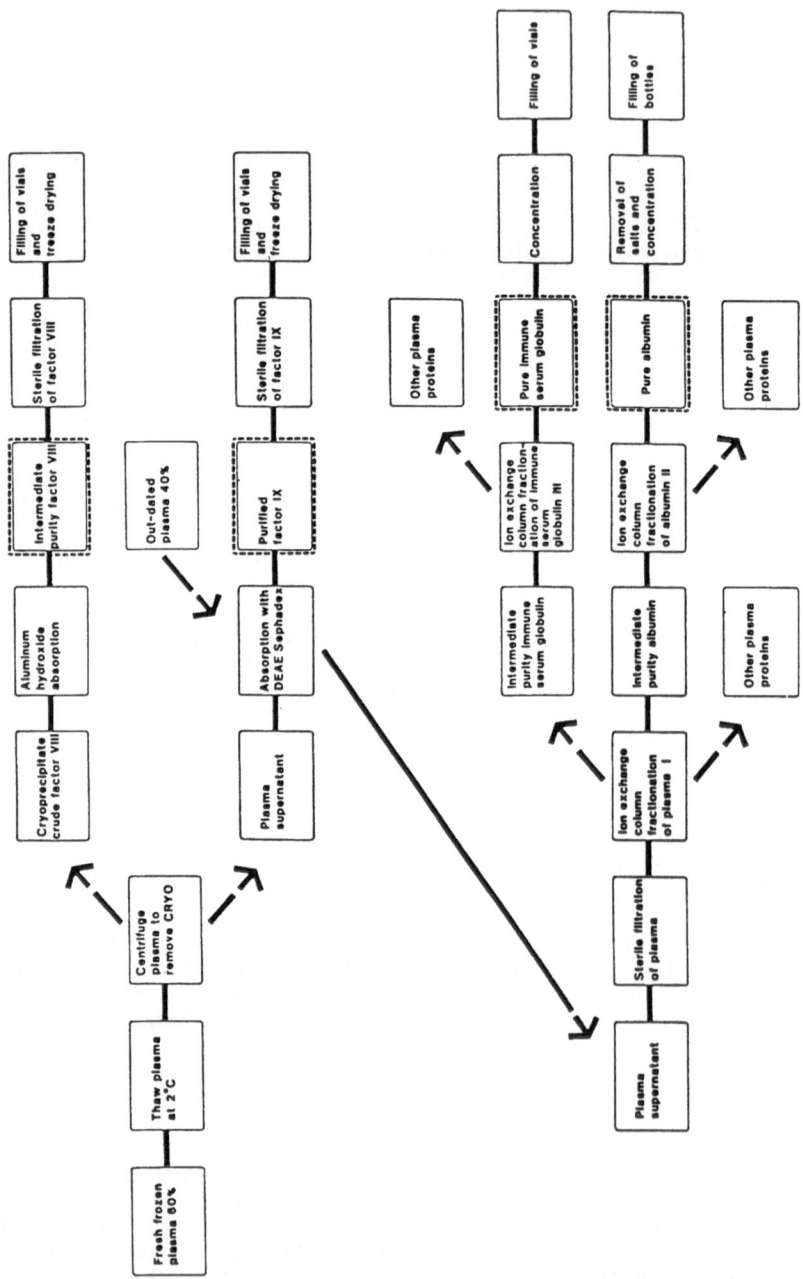

Figure 1. Schematic flow diagram of the Winnipeg Rh Institute
plasma fractionation process

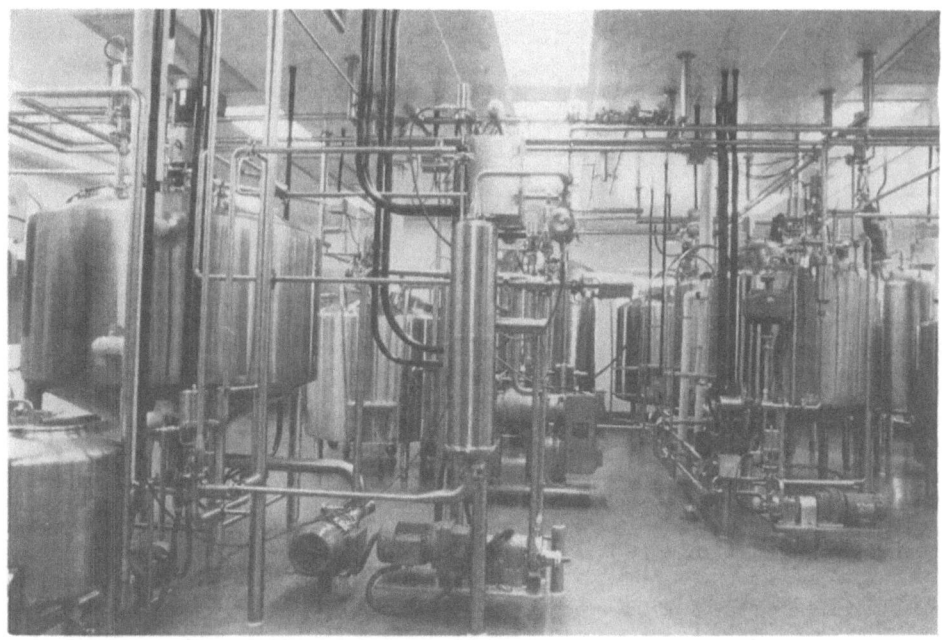

Figure 2. The "hard-piped" stainless steel process equipment for fractionation of 75,000 to 100,000 litres of plasma per year

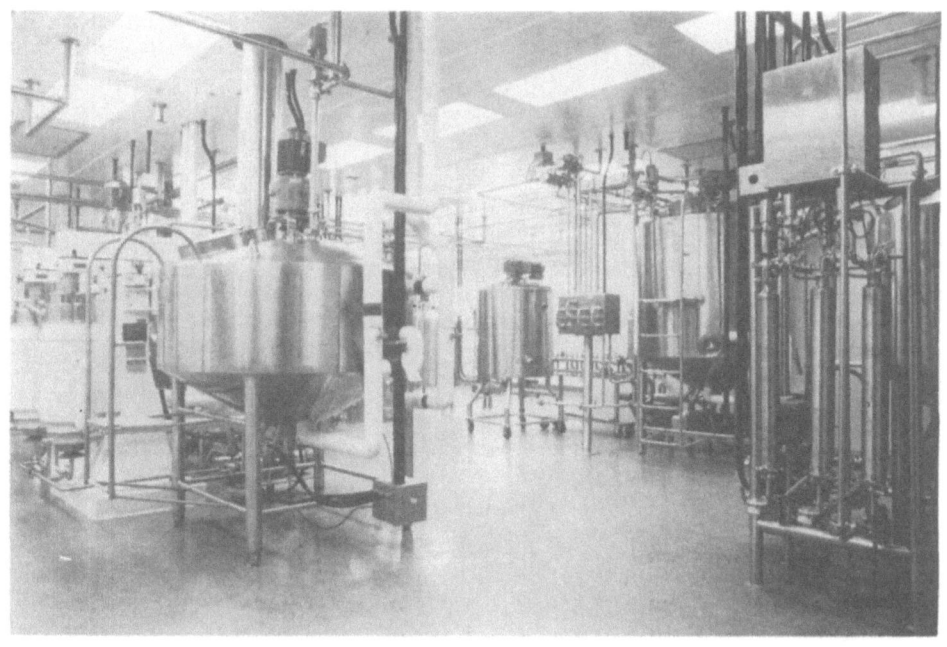

Figure 3. 800 litre plasma thaw thank for production of cryoprecipitate

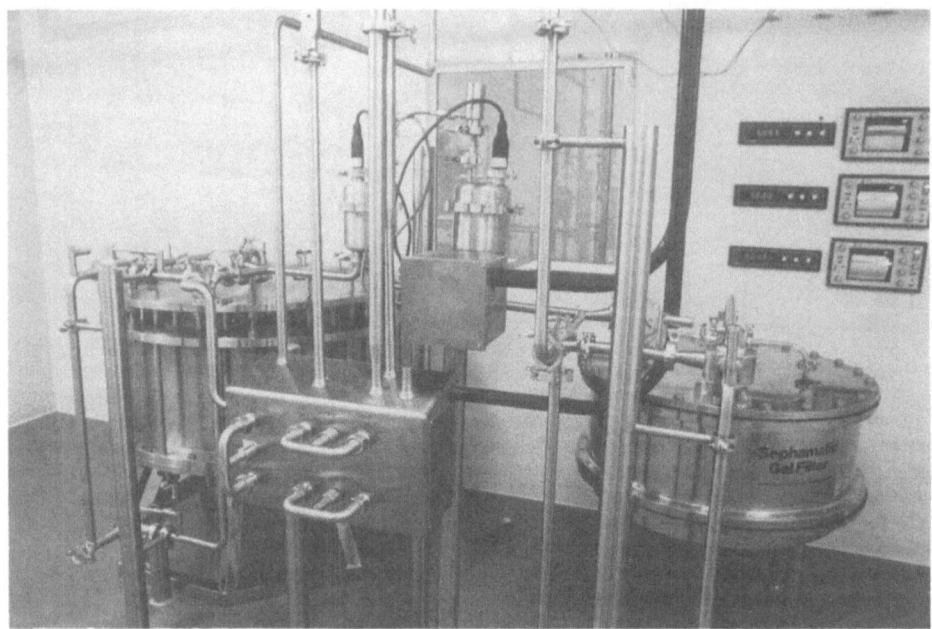

Figure 4. Two of the three colums; a 250 litre Amicon column
and a 150 litre Pharmacia column

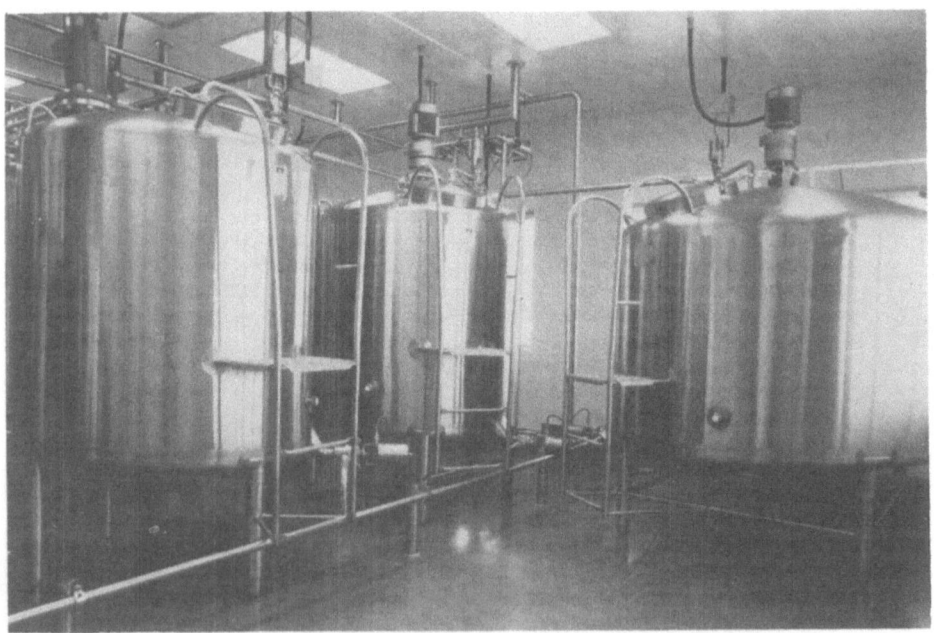

Figure 5. Three of the seven buffer holding tanks

Fresh frozen plasma is pooled from plastic donation bags into 800 litre volumes. The bags are dipped in liquid nitrogen to crack the plastic which is removed. The slugs of frozen plasma are dropped into a Guiloriver ice shaver which delivers the shavings into an 800 litre stainless steel thaw tank (fig. 3). Plasma is thawed under controlled temperatures to maintain the liquid plasma at 2°C. This results in the formation of cryoprecipitate. The thawed plasma is transferred via a positive displacement pump to AS26 Sharples centrifuges. The cryo-precipitate is collected in the bowls and the plasma supernatant is automatically transferred to a second tank for factor IX production. DEAE Sephadex is added to the cryo-poor plasma, incubated, allowed to settle, and the settled Sephadex is transferred into a small 15 litre sectional column for further purification of the factor IX prothrombin complex. Factor VIII in the cryoprecipitate is further purified by adsorption with aluminium hydroxide. The factor VIII- factor IX-deficient plasma is clarified by filtration with the aid of Celite followed by diafiltration with the Pelicon Ultra-filtration system to the pH and ionic strength of the first chromatography buffer.

Albumin and iv ISG are prepared from the dialyzed plasma by column chromatography with three ion exchangers; DEAE Sepharose CL-6B, DEAE Biogel A and CM Sepharose packed in columns of 250 litres (100 cm x 30 cm, stainless steel, Amicon), 150 litres (80 cm x 30 cm, stainless steel, Pharmacia), and 150 litres (630 cm x 50 cm, acrylic, Amicon), respectively (fig. 4). Diafiltered plasma is applied to a 230 litre stainless steel Amicon column packed with DEAE Sepharose with the aid of a positive displacement pump and a flowmeter. Acetate buffers are used to elute a crude IgG and a crude albumin fraction. The crude IgG is purified by ion exchange chromatography on a 150 litre Amicon column packed with DEAE Biogel. The crude albumin is purified on a 150 litre stainless steel Pharmacia column packed with CM Sepharose. Column effluent is monitored for UV absorbance, with ISCO monitors; pH, with Orion meters; and for conductivity, with Foxboro meters. Protein fractions are collected based on the UV absorbance at 280 nm. The seven buffers used in the separation process are prepared automatically by metering three stock solutions together with diluting water-for-injection (WFI) into holding tanks (fig. 5).

The entire stainless steel plasma fractionation equipment, including tanks, pipes, pumps, valves, sensors and monitors, is cleaned automatically with an eductor assisted CIP unit (fig. 6). The CIP unit circulates WFI through each of seven circuits. The CIP process involves the circulation of 57°C solutions of sodium hydroxide, phosphoric acid and hypochlorite, each followed by WFI rinses.

The entire plasma fractionation and CIP process is carried out automatically by a Modicon 584 Programmable Logic Controller through more than 600 input/output points, of which about 120 are analog devices (6). The control equipment is housed in a Main Control Panel (fig. 7) which also provides operator interface to the automated system via a control console. Automation is executed through a sequence of discrete automatic steps. The steps are initiated by operators via rotary switches, push buttons, machine tool switches, thumb wheel inputs and digital readouts. The operator begins the automatic sequence by turning the rotary switches to prescribed positions and then depressing the push button pilot lights which starts the process. The three chromatographic steps to produce iv ISG and albumin from plasma to the prescribed concentration are entirely automated without operator interruption.

Intermediate purity factor VIII of a specific activity of 800 units per gram is produced at an efficiency of 200-250 units per kilogram of

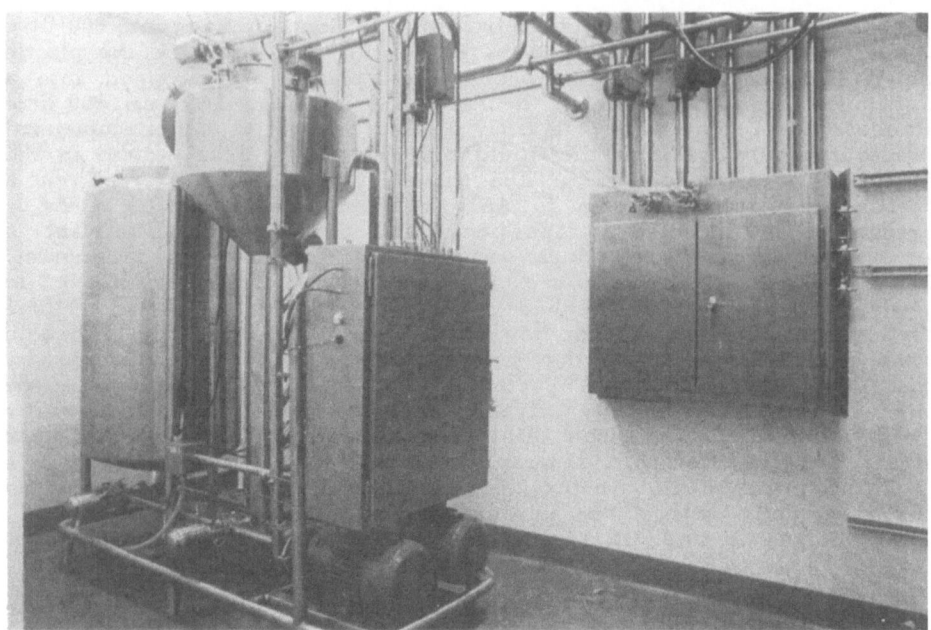

Figure 6. Clean-in-Place (CIP) unit

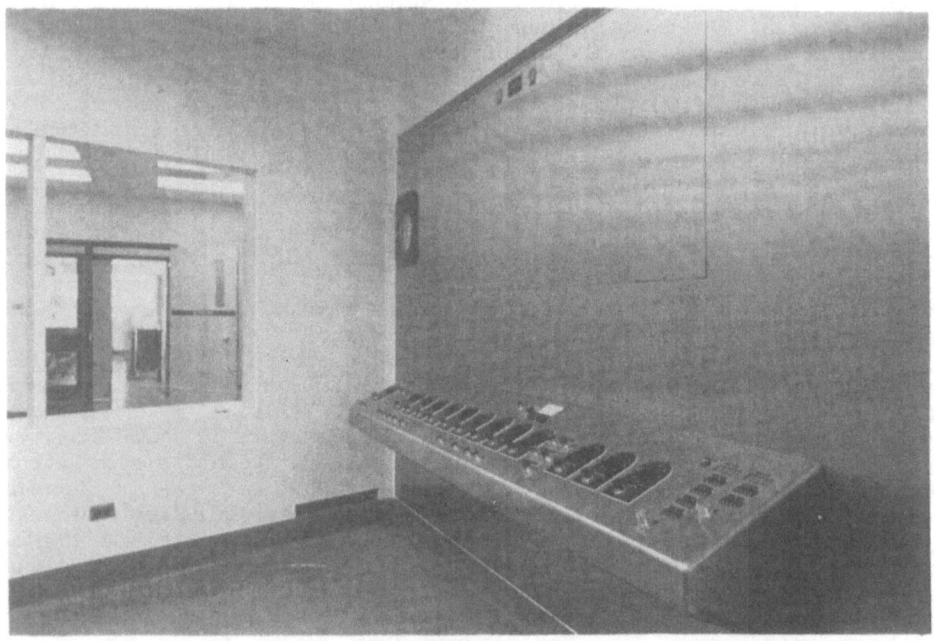

Figure 7. Main Control Panel which houses a Modicon Programmable
Controller system and provides operator interface with
automated process

plasma. Albumin of 98% purity, with less than 2% polymeric molecules, is recovered at a level of 80% to 85% efficiency. Immunoelectrophoretically pure ISG is recovered at 50% to 60% efficiency. It contains less than 1% aggregates, low anti-complement activity, no demonstrable IgM and less than 0.001% IgA. The biochemical characterization of albumin and ISG produced by the process has been reported previously (3-5).

SUMMARY

The Winnipeg Rh Institute has shown that an ion exchange chromatographic facility can be constructed with a capacity to fractionate at least 100,000 litres of plasma per year by an integrated system producing factor VIII, factor IX, iv ISG Albumin by a state-of-the-art automated, clean-in-place process, providing reliability, reduced labour and the documentation required for validation of a new pharmaceutical process.

ACKNOWLEDGEMENTS

The author thanks the entire staff at the Winnipeg Rh Institute who made the development of the facility described herein possible. A special note of appreciation is extended to H.W. Price, J. Rosolowich, C.E. Waskin, W.C.H. Bees and W.F. Grassler for their dedication to the project.

REFERENCES

1. Hoppe HH, Mester T, Hennig W, Krebs HJ. Prevention of Rh-immunization. Modified production of IgG anti-Rh for intravenous applications by ion exchange chromatography (IEC). Vox Sang 1973;25:308-16.
2. Friesen Ad, Bowman JM, Price HW. Column ion exchange preparation and characterization of an Rh immune globulin (WinRho) for intravenous use. J. Appl. Biochem. 1981;3:164-75.
3. Friesen AD, Bowman JM, Bees WCH. Column ion exchange chromatographic production of human immune globulins and albumin. In: Separation of Plasma Proteins, Curling JM ed. (Abstract presented at the 17th Congress of the International Society of Blood Transfusion), Budapest, 1982.
4. Friesen AD, Bowman JM, Bees WCH. Elution of HBsAg during ion exchange chromatographic production of albumin and immune serum globulin for intravenous use. Abstracts 18th Congress ISBT, S. Karger, Basel, 1984;161.
5. Friesen AD, Bowman JM, Bees WCH. Column ion exchange chromatographic production of human immune serum globulin for intravenous use. Vox Sang 1985;48:201-13.
6. Friesen AD. Programmable Logic Controller control of a blood fractionation process. Abstract Canadian Programmable Controllers Conference, IEEE, Montreal, 1984, 333.

LARGE SCALE CHROMATOGRAPHIC EXPERIMENTS FOR PLASMA FRACTIONATION

F. Haskó, K. Kristóf, M. Salamon, P. Dobó

INTRODUCTION

Recently several attempts have been made to find a fractionation procedure that replaces Cohn's cold alcohol technic. Curling et al. (1) developed a chromatographic fractionation system mainly for albumin and IgG. Using Gurling's results, we extended the system to produce other proteins, e.g. factor VIII and IX, antitrombin III, transferrin. The present paper summarizes the results of one and a half year of experimental production.

MATERIALS AND METHODS

Materials

All the chemicals used in the preparative experiments were of intravenous quality (Merck). The sterile water used was produced by a Reverse Osmosis (Millipore) system. The entire fractionation equipment (columns, monitors, tanks, gels) were from Pharmacia Fine Chemicals.

Plasma was separated from the blood of volunteer donors within 6 hours of the donation. Four to six units of plasma were pooled, frozen and kept at -30°C until use. After thawing, the cryoprecipitate was separated. Fifty liters of the cryosupernatant were used for every batch.

Factor IX

(protrombin complex concentrate = PCC) was produced according to Brummelhuis (2) (fig. 1). The coagulation factors were absorbed on DEAE-Sephadex in a stainless steal tank with a conical bottom. After removing the supernatant, the gel was washed three times with 5 l 0,01 M citrate + 0,2 M NaCl buffer. The PCC was eluted with 1 l 0,01 M citrate + 2 M NaCl buffer. The salt was removed by gel filtration on Sephadex G-25. After adding 3 U/ml Heparin the sterile filtered product was freeze dried.

Albumin

Fig. 2 shows the albumin procedure. The factor IX supernatant was desalted on a G-25 column to on ionic strength of I = 0,005 M. Then the so precipitated euglobulins were removed by centrifugation and filtration. The filtrate was chromatographed on a DEAE-Sepharose CL 6B FF column, eluting the IgG with pH 5.2, I = 0,025 M buffer, than the albumin with pH = 4.5, I = 0.025 M and at pH 4, I = 0.15 M the rest. The eluted albumin was chromatographed on the CM Sepharose CL 6B FF column. The bound albumin was eluted with pH 5.5, I = 0.11 M buffer and the rest with 0.4 M buffer. The second peak contains the antithrombin III. All buffers were Na acetate-acetic acid solutions. The eluate was concentrated by a Pelicon ultrafiltration system (Millipore) to a 6% protein concentration and then gel filtered on a Sephacryl S-200 column. Then the eluted albumin solution was again concentrated by ultrafiltration to 20% protein content. Finally, 0.005 M Na-caprylate was added to the end product, which was then sterile filtered and heat treated in bottles on 60°C for 10 hours.

IgG

was produced from the first DEAE Sepharose CL 6B FF peak (fig. 3). Solution was adjusted to pH = 6,5 I = 0.020 M by adding NaOH and diluting, then chromatographing again on a DEAE-Sepharose CL 6B FF column. The first IgG peak was eluted with the starting buffer, while the second, containing transferrin, with pH = 7.0 I = 1.0 M. The IgG peak was applied directly to the CM Sepharose CL 6B column. Washing began with the starting buffer (pH = 6.5 I = 0.02 M), repeated with 0.05 M NaCl. After adding albumin as a stabiliser, the solution was concentrated on a Pelicon ultrafilter to 5% protein content. At the end we added 10% glucose, sterile filtered and freeze dried.

All chromatographic steps (sample application, washing, eluting, equilibrating) have been controlled automatically, by Sephamatic C-2 units (Pharmacia).

Antithrombin III and transferrin

Some experiments have been carried out to adsorb antithrombin-III on heparin-Sepharose according to Wickerhauser (3). The transferrin containing peak was concentrated by ultrafiltration as a preliminary experiment.

Analytical methods

Protein determinations were made by the biuret method. The compositions of the fractions and the products were determined by acrylamid gel-, immuno-, and cellulose-acetate membrane electrophoresis. Protein polymers were measured by gel filtration on Superose column (Pharmacia).

Factor IX was tested by the "one stage" coagulation test. Complement activity of the IgG preparation was measured by the complement consumption method. Microbiological control of the process has involved sample-taking from each step and then culturing on agar-blood plates. In process pyrogenicity was tested by the limulus amoebyte lysate test. Pyrogenicity and toxicity of the endproducts were allways tested on rabbits and mice, as stated in Pharmacopeia. The quality control system is summerised in Table 1.

RESULTS

After testing the system for six months, we were ready for the pilot plant production. Our experiences are described below.

Factor IX

(Prothrombin complex concentrate). Table 2 depicts the results of PCC
production. It is obvious that all batches tested (84.03-84.13) are
pyrogenfree (tested on rabbits), although the limulus test shows mixed
results. This might have been caused either by the very high sensitivity
of the LAL test or by some unknown factors influencing the test. It is
also clear, that the yield must be improved; it varies between 22 and
69%. We also tested for factor IX content after each step, e.g. the
plasma after DEAE absorption, the washing solutions, but no loss of
factor IX was noted. It can be assumed that there are either unknown
artifacts during testing, or that the proteins are somehow damaged (by
proteases) and are partly deactivated during the process. This, of
course, requires further investigations.

Table 1. Quality control of plasma fractionation

Albumin

in-process control
  — determination of the protein content
  — pyrogenicity/LAL-test
  — microbiological
endproduct q.c.
  — determination of the protein content
  — protein composition
  — aggregate analysis
  — stability
  — sterility
  — pyrogenicity
  — toxicity

IgG

in-process control
  — determination of protein content
  — pyrogenicity/LAL-test
  — microbiological
endproduct q.c.
  — determination of protein content
  — protein composition
  — sterility
  — toxicity
  — pyrogenicity

PCC

in-process control
  — determination of protein content
  — measurement of the biological activity
  — microbiological
  — pyrogenicity/LAL-test
endproduct q.c.
  — testing of the biological activity
  — testing of activated factors
  — sterility
  — toxicity
  — pyrogenicity

108

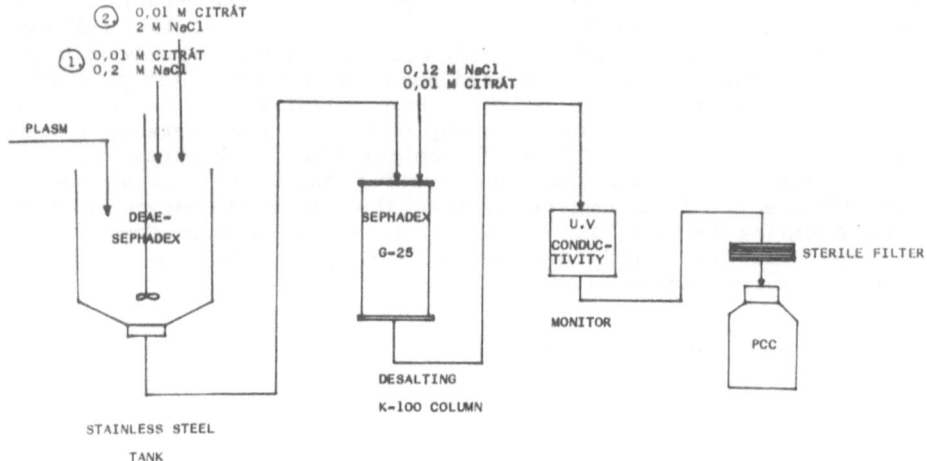

Figure 1. PCC Production Scheme

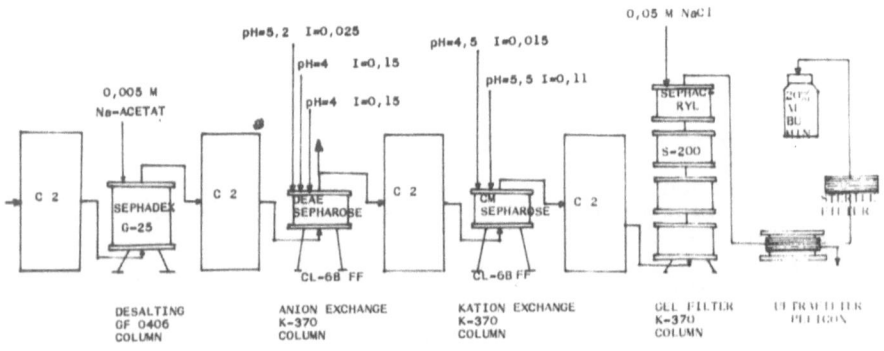

(C 2 = SEPHAMATIC CONTROLL BOX)

Figure 2. Albumin Production scheme

Table 2. Data on the production of factor IX concentrate

Batch No	Starting FactorIX U/ml	Plasma Volume ml	Product FactorIX U/ml	Product Volume ml	Yield %	Pyrogenicity Limulus	Pyrogenicity rabbit
84.15	0.78	50000	12	1760	54.15	+	
84.14	0.95	44000	15.8	1750	66	+	
84.13	0.82	44000	6	2520	34		−
84.12	0.91	45000	5.4	1900	22.8	+	−
84.11	0.95	44000	10	1850	45	−	−
84.10	1.1	40000	8.9	1900	41	−	−
84.09	0.92	48000	11	1900	47	+	−
84.08	0.9	44000	13	1780	58.4	−	−
84.07	1.2	44000	9	1720	29.3	+	−
84.06	1.0	35000	11	1740	54.7	−	−
84.04	0.6	50000	11.5	1800	69		−
84.03	0.7	50000	7	2400	48		−

Table 3. The result of albumin production

Batch no	Starting vol. l.	Plasma Protein g%	Product vol. ml	Product Protein g	Yield g/l	Pyrogenicity Limulus	Pyrogenicity rabbit
84.01	36	5.5	1267	733	20.3	−	−
84.02	50	5.1	1632	891	17.3	−	−
84.03	50	5.1	1632	905	18.1	+	−
84.04	48	5.25	1613	980	20.4	−	−
84.05	45	5.5	1584	832	18.5	+	−
84.06	44	5.6	1577	732	16.6	+	−
84.07	40	5.5	1408	252		−	−
84.08	44	4.6	1395	848	19.3	−	−
84.09	50	6.2	1984	864	17.3	−	−
84.10	44	5.15	1450	853	19.4	−	−
84.11	44	5.7	1605				−

Albumin

Table 3 illustrates the results of albumin production. All batches are pyrogenfree (tested by rabbits) but the limulus test — as in factor IX — shows different results. The mean yield of 17 g albumin per liter of plasma is insufficient. Albumin may have been lost because of failures in running the equipment. On the other hand, purity of the albumin was

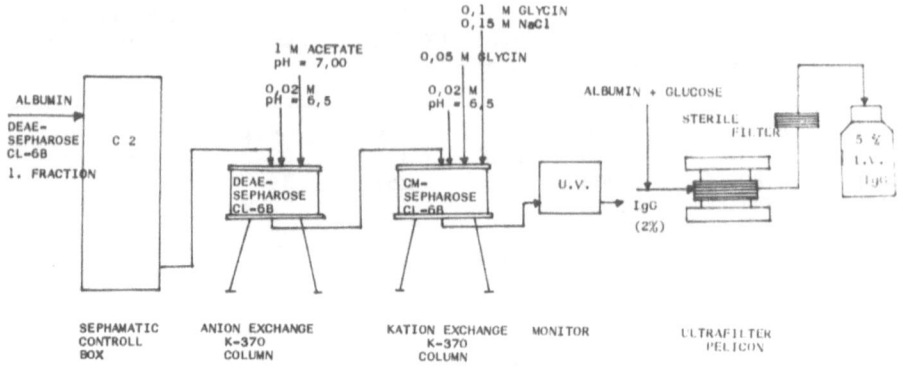

Figure 3. IV IgG Production Scheme

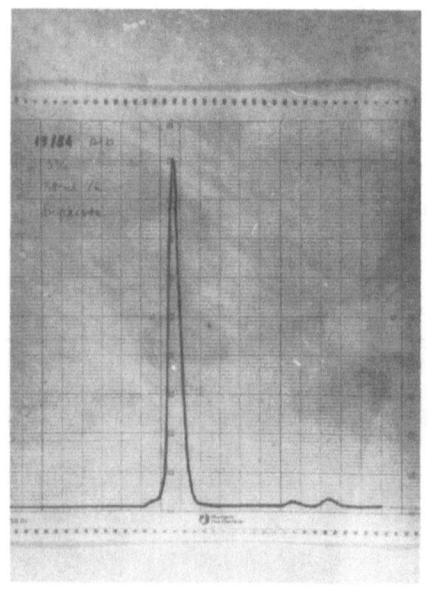

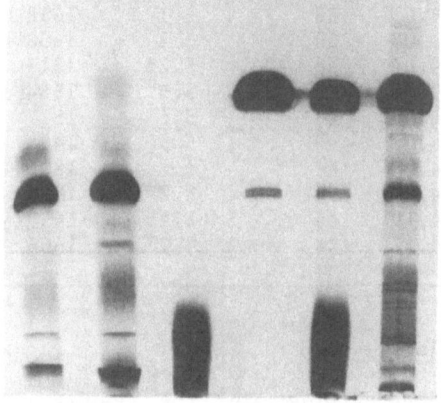

Figure 4. Elution diagram of albumin on Superose column.

Figure 5. Acrylamid gel electrophoresis pattern of fractions: (from left to right) after CM-Sepharose chromatography, after DEAE Sepharose, IgG, albumin, IV IgG stabilised with albumin, whole plasma.

Table 4. The results of intravenous IgG production

Batch no	Starting volume (1)	Product volume (1)	IgG protein (%)	Pyrogenicity limu- lus	rabbit	Anti compl. activity	
84.01	50	0.8	3	−	−	0	
84.02	48.8	3.4	5	+	−	28.5	*
84.03	35	2.4	5	−	−	16.8	*
84.05	39	0.5	5	±	+	0	
84.06	44	2.0	5	−	−	12.5	
84.07	44	3.1	5	+	−	-2.5	
84.08	50	3.9	5	−	−	-6.0	
84.09	50	4.0	2.3	−	−	−	

* By the use of $0.2\,\mu m$ Millipore cartridge before the 2nd DEAE column, the anticomplement activity became very high, probably caused by the sheare effect of high pressure filtration.

outstanding, containing very few polymers (fig. 4). Stability of the albumin solution was not always acceptable. In batch 9 and 10 we observed precipitates during pasteurisation. The product had a green colour, confirming O'Riordan's observation (4).

The reason for this may be the presence of billiverdin, that was found very strongly bound to the albumin. Theoretically, billiverdin can be removed by $0.055\ M\ H_2O_2$, UV-irradiation or by caprilic acid precipitation, but it is still an open question whether it has to be removed at all.

Intravenous IgG

Results of the few experiments made with IgG are shown in Table 4. The product was pyrogenic only once (tested on rabbits), all other experiments showed to pyrogen. The low yield needs further investigation. Anticomplement activity was high only in the 2 batches. This was caused by high pressure filtration before the CM step. It also became obvious that the product must be freeze dried. In liquid state aggregates may form, and this may result in anticomplement activity. The purity of this product is shown in fig. 5. Subclass distribution is shown in Table 5.

Microbial decontamination

The equipment has been placed in a clean room, with filtered air $(0,45\ \mu m)$. The personnel entering the room must change their clothes and wear caps. They also wear masks when working with plasma in open tanks. Every small pool of plasma is tested for bacterial contamination before processing. Only sterile plasma is used. Our recently developed decontamination methodology is summarised in Table 6.

Table 5. Subclass distribution of IV IgG batches

Batch No	IgG1	IgG2	IgG3	IgG4
84.01	71.3	22.0	6.3	1.4
84.02	66.5	25.2	6.7	1.6
84.03	75.3	17.7	6.1	0.9
84.04	71.3	20.6	6.9	1.2
84.05	72.4	19.9	6.4	1.3
84.06	67.3	24.8	7.1	0.8
84.07	68.0	24.7	6.5	0.8
84.08	70.7	21.2	7.1	1.0
mean	70.4	22.0	6.6	1.0
WHO ref. plasma	60.0	29.4	6.5	4.1

Clinical application and trials

Factor IX produced by our system has been in clinical use for some time. Clinical investigations of the batches of albumin gave satisfactory results.

Cost

Table 7 shows the total cost of the products in Hungarian currency and the cost distribution of the components. The significant factors in arriving at these figures have been plasma price, chemicals, gels and salaries.

DISCUSSION

The experiments lasting for 18 months have proven the applicability of the chromatographic technic. These products meet the requirements of the pharmacopeia. Because of the very mild fractionation, the proteins remain in their natural state as it is stated by Martinache et al (5) in the case of albumin. The IgG is not reduced, digested by enzymes or treated with chemicals. The IgG subclass distribution is only slightly different from the normal plasma. The complement consumption is low, indicating suitability of the product for intravenous use.

While the decontamination methodoly developed by us contributes to pyrogenfree products, the economy of the system needs further development. All yields must be increased, including the yield of factor IX. We are also aware of the fact that the yields of albumin with 17 g/liter plasma and the IgG's with about 3 g/liter plasma are worse as compared to Cohn's method, or the rivanol method used in our specific IgG production. Yield naturally effects production costs. If the yield can be increased to 25 g albumin/liter plasma, then the production cost would decrease to 37 Ft/g, i.e. to half of the present cost.

Table 6. Decontamination system

Gel or equipment	decontaminant	exp. time	storage
Sephadex G-25	0.5 M NaOH	30 min	0.25 M NaOH
DEAE Sepharose CL 6B	1.0 M NaOH	3 h	
CM Sepharose CL 6B	1.0 M NaOH	3 h	1.0 M CH$_3$COOH
Sephacryl S-200	0.2 M NaOH	48 h	0.01 M NaOH
CEPA-centrifuge	washing + autoclaving		
Ultrafilter	0.5 M NaOH wash and backwash		1 M CH$_3$COOH

All buffers are made from fresh RO-water. The buffers are sterile filtered (Durapore 0,3 m Cartridge, Millipore)

Table 7. Production cost of plasma proteins

			Cost distribution in %				
Product	Plasma	Chemicals	Gels	Filters + cons.	Salary	Q.C.	Total cost
Albumin	41	20	15	2	20	2	60 Ft/g
IV IgG	34	25	15	3	20	3	150 Ft/g
PCC	20	37	6	11	20	6	1 Ft/U
Anti-D IgG	62	12	7	2	11	4	1 Ft/μg

Currently one batch is run per week. Columns must be decontaminated after every batch, however, to effectively remove the decontaminating agent sodium hydroxide, a larger amount of buffer (sterile water, chemicals, filters) is needed.

Running two or more batches per week will require a more continuous work, which may bring about a decrease in the specific consumption of chemicals. The introduction of new products, e.g. transferrin, antithrombin III and factor VIII should also lower some of the specific costs.

In summary, using chromatography for the production of therapeutic plasma proteins is rather advantageous. The products are of good quality and the sytem can be easily extended for the production of other proteins. To exploit all of its potential advantages, however, further extensive studies will be required.

REFERENCES

1. Curling JM. Methods of Plasma Protein Fractionation. Academic Press, London U.K. 1980.
2. Brummelhuis HGJ. Preparation of the prothrombin complex. In: Methods of Plasma Protein Fractionation. Academic Press London U.K. 1980.

3. Wickerhauser M, Williams C, Mercer J. Developments of large scale fractionation methods. VII Preparation of antithrombin III concentrate. Vox Sang 1979;36:281-93.
4. O'Riordan: Personal communication.
5. Martinache L, Henon MP, Goudemand M. Large scale albumin fractionation by chromatography. In: Separation of Plasma Proteins. Curling JM ed, Pharmacia, Uppsala 1983.

DISCUSSION

Moderators: J.K. Smith, H.G.J. Brummelhuis

L.V. Milner (Durban):

Dr. Over, concerning homogenous freezing of plasma: As long as the plasma is frozen within three hours, that is adequate. Or must it be quicker than that?

J. Over:

That is a problem we will have to study. Unfortunately, we did not investigate a freezing time between fifteen minutes and three hours. Fifteen minutes was optimal, while three hours gave poorer results.

L.V. Milner:

The problem is that it is very difficult to do in practice on a large scale.

J. Over:

It depends on what you call a large scale. For instance, what has been put into use a few months ago at our institute is freezing by means of nitrogen vapour of -70°C, not -100°C, as was shown; -70°C allows a freezing time of 20 minutes. I am not fully acquainted with the figures, but I guess we can freeze 200 bags at one time in 20 minutes, or perhaps 300 in one box.

L.V. Milner:

Have you any idea what it costs per bag to freeze under those conditions?

J.A. Loos:

One litre of liquid nitrogen costs 20 cents in our country and one needs 1.5 litre of nitrogen to freeze 300 ml of plasma below -30°C. We freeze 20 units at a time at -70°C within 25 minutes in a cabinet with the vapour of boiling liquid nitrogen.

C.Th. Smit Sibinga:

Dr. Over, what makes the lyophilisation so different compared to what Dr. Foster has experienced over the years? What is it in the pore glass method which yields finally these threads, and gives you the problem?

J. Over:

Actually, I forgot to mention that at first we concentrated by an 8% PEG step only, which led to very heavy precipitates after lyophilisation and dissolution. Protein analysis suggested it to be mainly fibrinogen.

A 5% step which removes fibrinogen seems to solve the problem but not in 100% of the cases. That is our problem now. I think it is mainly fibrinogen which is unstable. I do not know the reason for this. I do not think it is the lyophilisation process. We analysed the strands being formed and there is also some fibronectin in them. I think the main problem is fibrinogen.

C.Th. Smit Sibinga:

You did not show any specific step for removing the vast amount of fibronectin. It is usually fibronectin which causes the problem during ultrafiltration of a finished product like FVIII, which may lead to thread formation during lyophilisation.

J. Over:

I am not sure. I think both proteins are very difficult to handle, both in ultrafiltration and in lyophilisation. We did not include a step to remove fibronectin.

F. Peetoom:

Dr. Smit Sibinga, I felt that you made a philosophical case for self-sufficiency. I just wonder if that is an end in itself or whether you have indications that the reduction of loss or increase of recovery, or the safety aspects, or the economy (which is very important these days) are part of your goals. What evidence do you have to give substance to the self-sufficiency notion in (sub)regionalising the production of proteins. I would like to hear more facts about it than just the philosophy, which in itself I think may be valid.

C.Th. Smit Sibinga:

One of the statements made this morning by Dr. Gunson is that, for a number of countries, depending on the size and the technology available, it does not make sense to go for national fractionation facilities. Therefore, other means should be developed to achieve that final finished product: Albumin, gammaglobulin, and others like FVIII. Dr. Gunson pointed to the industry. I pointed to more regionalisation. What I meant by "strength through combined regional effort" is on a smaller scale. Through smaller pools the safety could improve. Smaller scales usually have better yields than larger scales.

Economically, one could more easily reach and support that self-sufficiency goal than through sending in plasma massively to the large-scale types of procedures. It is something which might come along. This is being put in practice in a number of countries, not only in Europe, but specifically outside Europe. I have visited quite a number of countries in the last couple of years, and I was surprised to see that even in small operations like in Yugoslavia, column chromatography gets off the ground and moves into fulfilling the prophecy of becoming self-suffiecient. They have had a major decision to make: Should we go for national fractionation or simply regionalise? They have chosen, for the time being, for regionalisation.

A similar thing is happening to a certain extent in South Africa, at the moment. There is a major centre in Durban, but there are a number of other centres in South Africa doing smaller-scale fractionation, producing albumin and gammaglobulins on a regional basis. I could add a number of other countries to the list, i.e. Brazil and Hungary.

F. Peetoom:

Would you consider this development as an experimental approach to finding a new way? I feel that there may still be some questions as to whether this new cottage-industry approach — which, by the way, is evolving in other industries, and appears to be very advantageous because there is much less capital investment required and much faster response to changes in technology than when it is localised in one large centralised industry which would have to make major costly changes — is advantageous. I think there are advantages, but it is my opinion, from what I hear, that it is in transition and still being evaluated rather than being able to say that this is the end of the line. I can see that there might be a marriage between small scale treatment and a centralised process, which would combine different advantages. There may be a different solution, and this is just one current direction that is being explored. Is my conclusion correct?

C.Th. Smit Sibinga:

This is definitely not the end of the line, but one of the steps along the line. I definitely believe in a marriage in this connection. But these techniques as they have come along this line certainly have a meaning: they have something to contribute. In the countries which I named, this was basically getting off the ground at a certain point in time instead of wasting time and hard currency to import the necessary products for clinical purposes.

H.H. Gunson:

Can I follow this up, Dr. Smit Sibinga? Perhaps I missed it, but I did not understand just exactly what volume size of pools you were dealing with. I agree your concept of donors is right, but what is the actual volume that you put through the process?.

C.Th. Smit Sibinga:

I am shifting away from the definition of pool size, because when we speak about volumes we speak about a different entity. These techniques like column chromatography run, for instance, off 50 litres per week, which is entirely different from what is done in a major fractionation centre. The controlled pore glass chromotography can be run at very small volumes, even smaller than 50 litres per week. The heparin double cold precipitation method deals with volumes per batch off 3 to 6 litres.

H.H. Gunson:

This is the point that I was trying to take this morning. If you are dealing with a pool size of 3 to 6 litres, it is extraordinarily difficult to often fulfill all regulatory requirements. How are you able to accomplish this with respect to that? Because otherwise you do it at the expense of a large proportion of the yield of the batch.

C.Th. Smit Sibinga:

That is definitely true. One of the major aims which we have set in our heparin double cold precipitation principle is, that it should not interfere with routine bloodbanking technology (1) I think we have accomplished that.
   Another aim is in cost effectiveness: One should initiate the concept that more than one product should be made out of the starting material, otherwise it will not be cost effective. If you waste the red cells, you load all the costs on the plasma, and eventually on the plasma proteins. So it is a matter of balance.

J.K. Smith:

Dr. Over, it was intriguing that the reduction in ionic strenght by dialysis against distilled water improved the efficiency of cryoprecipitation. You must have given some thought to exploitation of this possibility. I wonder if you could share any of these ideas with us?

J. Over:

There were many thoughts, actually. I do not see a quick way to introduce it on a large scale, because the bags are frozen on the spot at the blood collection facility and the whole thing should be done before freezing.

F. Peetoom:

I worked for a while at Hyland Laboratories. I remember when I got there in 1968, they had found indeed a doubling of potency by dialysis

1. Smit Sibinga CTh, Welbergen H, Das PC, Griffin B. High-yield method of production of freeze-dried purified factor VIII by blood banks. Lancet 1981;ii:449-50.

against water. It is a long time ago, so I do not remember all the details, but it has not been put into a manufacturing process, because there was something with the stability of that dialysed product. I wonder how much study you have done with this particular component to see that it is a stable FVIII molecule that will recover well, that will assay in both direct and indirect, two-stage and one-stage techniques for the same potency, so that there are some indicators that you are really working with a satisfactory molecule of adequate stability?

J. Over:

We have not done so.

H.G.J. Brummelhuis (Amsterdam):

Dr. Curling, may I ask two or three questions? The first one is concerning the introduction of this arginine-sepharose: What is the background of this introduction?

J.M. Curling (Uppsala):

It is only for the enzyme activity; to reduce the plasminogen and the PKA activity. What we have done is to look at the use of Aerosil, as practised in one or two places, especially its use in the centre in Minnesota, who are preparing IVIgG. We do not like the use of Aerosil, because of presence of traces of silica in the final products, as far as we can determine. There also are losses of IgG, and disturbance of the subclass distribution. But by avoiding the use of Aerosil, in this method at least, we can produce an IgG which has the subclasses in almost exactly the same ratio as they occur in the plasma. So, that is really our background to looking for an alternative, as well as the difficulty of using this voluminous powder in production. It is not an easy material to handle, as you well know.

H.G.J. Brummelhuis:

The second question concerns the high value prekallikreïne mentioned.

J.M. Curling:

That is what we are planning to do with this immobilised benzamidine. We do not yet understand the mechanism of it, but we have the privileged position being able to test different immobilised protease scavengers.

F. Peetoom:

Dr. Middleton, did you mention what your final recovery was, through this process?

S.H. Middleton (Wrexham):

Through the process with human plasma, it is about 30%, but that is not going through filtration and freeze-drying.

J.K. Smith:

In connection with removal of HBsAg, I have two questions. One, whether you have quantitated the removal in terms of the number of log removal. Secondly, whether the extensive washing used for that experiment would be compatible with the yield you have obtained in normal practice?

S.H. Middleton:

The washing is the same amount as we normally use. We normally wash down to protein baseline, and that is what we were using to monitor the experiments.

We have not looked at it in terms of log removal — the amount of hepatitis B antigen that we were using ranged from levels that are below detection, about 0.2 nanograms. The detection level is 0.5, so that is equivalent to what you would possibly have in a pool of plasma. It goes up to very high levels, 5 nanograms and higher. In HBV we added 1 milligram per ml of antigen, which is very high. We are using an assay that detected it down to 3 picograms per ml, and could not detect it in the eluate.

J. Over:

I noticed that the recovery of FVIII in this step with the monoclonal antibody against FVIII:C was 80%. Has it been tried on plasma?

S.H. Middleton:

Yes. The purity that you get is not terribly good and the recovery is not as good as that.

J. Over:

I wonder whether this monoclonal antibody could be used to extract FVIII:C from plasma for producing a concentrate.

S.H. Middleton:

The elution conditions from the FVIII:C antibody involve polyethylene glycol, and fairly severe conditions, although the FVIII:C you get off is active. This is always a problem with monoclonal purification.

W.G. van Aken (Amsterdam):

Dr. Lake, the figures you have presented to us have certain margins. I was interested in the figures you presented on FVIII, because you said that $ 1,000,000 could be counted in profits by 1990. Is that taking into account the fact that the FVIII can be administered not only by the intravenous way, but perhaps may be taken orally?

W.C. Lake (Deerfield):

No, it does not.

W.G. van Aken:

So, your figures refer only to intravenous administration?

W.C. Lake:

Yes. I was simply speculating on the basis of the intravenous use of the product. That assumes introduction of the product in 1989, at the earliest. I think the figures for FVIII are optimistic estimates, but not overly optimistic. We will be able to make a much better estimate in the next 12 months as to whether those may be the true time frames that we are talking about for the introduction of that product.

F. Peetoom:

In the last statement, you observed that the appearance of FVIII from recombinant source might or may be favourably impact on the progress with recombinant albumin. I wondered why you chose the words 'may or might'. I feel that it is very significant to remove the income from FVIII from source plasma cost recovery. I think it is tremendously destructive for the whole plasma industry. Did you deliberately choose the words 'may or might'?

W.C. Lake:

Yes, I did. I think that the price dynamics are so complex. There was some discussion earlier about whether or not one should talk about some certain fraction driving the plasma fractionation market or not.
What will happen, if a FVIII product appears: There is a certain standard basic cost to processing plasma. If you take the FVIII portion out of that, then the cost is going to be redistributed among the remaining products. How it is going to be redistributed is not clear. It may be all placed on albumin. That is certainly the most logical place to put it, probably, because that is the place that can best handle it and still allow you to produce the other products. If you make that shift and then try to recalculate and determine whether or not it now becomes economically attractive to build a large recombinant DNA manufacturing facility, is still a very difficult process to speculate on.

C.Th. Smit Sibinga:

Dr. Friesen, two short questions. One is: What is the total processing capacity in terms of litres? Secondly: What is the cost of starting this plant?

A.D. Friesen (Winnipeg):

I will answer your second question first. The total cost of the equipment was $ 2.6 million (Can.) — or about $ 2 million (US). The facility cost was also $ 2.6 million (Can.) or about $ 2 million US. The plant was originally designed with a capacity of about 75,000 litres per year. That is, the capacity to process one batch of 800 litres on Monday and another batch of 800 litres on Wednesday. The weekly schedule to process Monday and Wednesday was based on estimated flow rates for the 200 litre Sepharose columns. During start-up, we discovered that the actual flow rates were higher than estimated. We can now process 800 litres through the chromatographic step in less than 24 hours which provides a significantly greater capacity. We are still not sure how much we will be able to process at full capacity, but we are limited to an 800 litre pool by the size of the tank and at 4 batches per week we estimate the ultimate capacity without modification could be over 100,000 litres per year.

H.G.J. Brummelhuis:

May I ask Dr. Curling to comment on the green albumin?

J.M. Curling:

Green albumin is not only an Irish disease. It comes from all sorts of places. We have tried to do some studies on this.

First of all I would like to say that it is not really valid what colour it is, although it seems to be in all studies that have been done. All the infusions into patients of albumin which is green were without any effect whatsoever. So, I suggest perhaps a change in the pharmacopea statement would be more appropriate.

However, the colour seems to us to depend on how fresh the plasma is when you start fractionating, and how long you have stored the albumin preparation before you issue it. It seems to be an effect of light, you can keep the plasma a long time in a freezing room before you fractionate it. It is quite O.K. if it comes out yellow to brown if it is very old plasma. If it is fresh plasma, it is bound to be greenish. I can only recommend that you use old plasma, and then you store your final products for some time in the light, not in the dark.

H.G.J. Brummelhuis:

Maybe, you could add a very low amount of vitamin C to your buffers during fractionation.

J.M. Curling:

Yes, it helps. I think Dr. Haskó has some experience of that, but we do not want to introduce any more chemicals into processing, if we do not have to.

F. Haskó (Budapest):

We made a lot of experiments with the green albumin, because our clinicians were anxious. At first we tried some UV-radiation, but we found out that it is bound very strongly. It can be done by exchange chromatography, but we have not decided whether to remove it or not. That is a question for the future.

III. Safety aspects

PRESERVATION OF STRUCTURE AND FUNCTION DURING ISOLATION OF HUMAN PLASMA PROTEINS

J.J. Morgenthaler, U.E. Nydegger

INTRODUCTION

Purified plasma proteins have been used therapeutically ever since they became available, thanks to the pioneering work of Cohn and his associates in the forties. Fractionation with ethanol is now so well established in the trade and the advantages of this precipitant are so obvious that its use is rarely questioned. It is becoming increasingly clear, however, that all separation methods may, in some way, impose stress on the proteins isolated. At the very least, even the gentlest isolation method will remove a protein from its normal surroundings and place it in a solution where the protective influences by other proteins and low molecular mass solutes is lost.

For many years, the main product of plasma fractionation was albumin; the most important function of this protein is the preservation of oncotic pressure, a property which is proportional to the number of molecules present in solution. Manufacturers were therefore mostly concerned with achieving good recoveries and avoiding the formation of polymers. Oncotic activity was measured, but it is obviously a poor indicator for structural integrity of the molecule.

Later on, coagulation factors became important plasma derivatives, and the situation reversed: coagulation assays are — though hardly of outstanding precision — readily available to all fractionators. The aim now was to recover as many "activity units" as possible from each liter of plasma. The actual protein mass was rarely measured, in part because it is very low: coagulation factors have a very high specific activity. Fractionators were not too different from the biochemists who isolate an enzyme from any suitable source and publish tables showing recoveries and purification factors, but worry little about the fate of the "lost" activity. However, in the case of plasma proteins used intravenously, this "lost" activity might be of paramount importance to the patient, who could be faced with unwanted neo-antigens.

In view of its great practical and economic importance one might expect a great deal of knowledge concerned with possible changes occurring during plasma fractionation; this is, however, not the case. Extensive searches of the literature revealed only very few publications dealing with this subject. The best currently available evidence which indicates that plasma proteins undergo little changes during fractionation is their long-standing record of efficacy and safety. Nevertheless, it might be important to develop better ways of assessing the functional and structural integrity of isolated plasma proteins. This is now a particularly timely task, since we will be faced soon with genetically engineered proteins whose complete identity with human plasma proteins will have to be demonstrated. A major problem encountered in all these studies obviously consists in finding a suitable standard.

This review is not comprehensive; we merely try to illustrate a few points with examples either found in the literature or from our own experience.

SURVEY OF FRACTIONATION METHODS

Separation methods for proteins have been categorized as follows (1):
- methods based on differtential solubility (precipitation methods based on changes in ionic concentration of pH or mediated by organic solvents, polymers, metal ions, organic cations, anionic substances; partition in multiphasic systems)
- methods based on differential interactions with solid media (surface adsorption; ion exchange and affinity chromatography; separation by exclusion chromatography or semipermeable membranes)
- methods based on differential interactions with physical fields (centrifugation, electrophoresis, differential thermal denaturation).

Only a few of these procedures are used in commercial plasma fractionation. The following discussion therefore focusses on the technically important methods.

Precipitation

Inspite of the rapid progress in, e.g., chromatographic methods, precipitation is still the most commonly used separation method in plasma fractionation. This is not only due to the fractionator's conservatism, but also to the simplicity of the methods involved. Besides other advantages, precipitation avoids the large increases in volume which normally plague chromatographic methods.

Organic solvents

Ethanol is the most widely used solvent. Its main advantages are its chemical inertness, low toxicity, volatility, low price, and availability; it can easily be reclaimed from waste fractions. Since it depresses the freezing point of water, fractionation can be carried out at low temperatures; together with the inherent bacteriostatic properties of ethanol, low temperatures help to inhibit the growth of micro-organisms (2). Disadvantages of ethanol are its possible negative effects on protein structure and its poor specificity as a precipitating agent.

Polymers

The usefulness of poly(ethylene glycol) (PEG) as a precipitating agent has been known for a long time (3); more recently, other organic polymers (poly-vinylpyrrolidone; Ficoll; albumin) have been tested as precipitants (4). PEG presumably has no denaturing effect on proteins, even at room temperature. Fractionation may therefore be carried out without investing in expensive cooling equipment. A complete fractionation scheme, based on PEG precipitation, has been proposed (5). The most common methods for purification of factor VIII use PEG precipitation (6).

Compared with ethanol fractionation, where both the precipitant and the low temperature help to control bacterial growth, PEG fractionation is at a disadvantage. Additionally, removal of PEG from the end product is not yet satisfactorily solved; although it is probably non-toxic (7) and has been well tolerated by the hemophiliacs over many years, its absence in the final product would still be desirable. Unspecificity as a precipitating agent has to be added to the list of PEG's drawbacks.

Other reagents

Salts, and particularly ammonium sulfate, have been used for a century as protein precipitants. Other useful reagents include rivanol (2-ethoxy-6,9-diamino-acridine) and caprylic acid (8). Although they probably do little harm to most proteins, these chemicals are often toxic and have to be removed from products intended for intravenous use. Additionally, safe and environmentally acceptable disposal of these reagents could be a problem. This might explain why fractionation schemes based on these reagents never became very popular.

Chromatography

Gel chromatography

Gel chromatography has virtually no denaturing effect on proteins and almost 100% quantitative recoveries can be expected; it should therefore be ideally suitable for the isolation of sensitive proteins. Unfortunately, the protein masses that can be handled by reasonably sized columns are small, and the dilution of the sample cannot be neglected. This method is therefore not much used in plasma fractionation, with one notable exception: removal of ethanol and salts from albumin precipitates can be carried out safely and efficiently with Sephadex G-25. The dilution factor is well below 2 and the process can be fully automatized (9).

Ion exchange chromatography

Some distortions of the protein molecules might occur while they are adsorbed on the ion exchange matrix; the relatively high salt concentrations and/or pH-values diverging from neutrality that are required for desorption could also affect protein structure. Nevertheless, ion exchange chromatography is considered a gentle separation method. Schemes that allow purification of the most important plasma proteins have been published (10-12). Unfortunately, comprehensive schemes are usually rather complex, and they often have to make use of other techniques as well (e.g., precipitation), so that the inherent advantages of ion exchange chromatography are at least partially lost.

Factor IX (rather the "Prothrombin Complex") is commonly prepared by adsorption on DEAE-Sephadex, followed by elution with high salt concentrations (13).

Affinity chromatography

Affinity chromatography is a highly selective purification method; stress on the protein molecule is probably moderate, particularly when immobilized natural substrates can be used as ligands. Problems might arise when the specific and sometimes very strong binding between protein and ligand has to be broken during elution. When enzymes are isolated with the help of immobilized substrates, elution is usually achieved with excess dissolved substrate. Subsequently, the protein has to be separated from its substrate.

Unfortunately, few suitable ligands are available for the isolation of plasma proteins. A notable exception is fibronectin, which can easily be isolated by affinity chromatography on immobilized gelatin (14). In the first publication, elution of fibronectin was achieved with urea; this not only introduces an undesirable chemical into the protein solution; it also (probably reversibly) destroys the protein's secondary structure. Later publications demonstrated that elution was also possible under less drastic conditions. Using a ligand with a slightly lowered affinity for fibronectin we showed that elution is possible by slightly lowering the pH and raising the temperature; both measures are easily reversible and leave no trace in the protein solution (15).

Ultrafiltration

Ultrafiltration membranes are availble with different nominal pore sizes; they are, however, useless for the separation of proteins from each other, since their behavior is influenced by the other components in solution. On the other hand, ultrafilters have been succesfully used for the concentration of isolated plasma proteins, e.g., albumin (16). Although the method is gentle, shear forces may cause some problems.

FACTORS WITH POSSIBLE ADVERSE EFFECTS

Ethanol

It is generally accepted that ethanol denatures proteins; lipoproteins seem to be particularly susceptible in this respect and can be irreversibly denatured by ethanol. However, fractionators also believe that carefully controlled conditions, and specially low temperatures, will offset any untoward effect ethanol might have on plasma proteins (2). Nevertheless, this is not always the case, as has been demonstrated a long time ago with immunoglobulins.

Schultze and collaborators (17) noticed that immunoglobulins prepared by alcohol fractionation according to Cohn's method resolve in the ultracentrifuge into a major peak with a relative molecular mass of 156,000 and a minor peak with a relative molecular mass of about 300,000. The second peak apparently contains immunoglobulin dimers. In contrast, the dimer peak was not observed when other immunoglobulin fractions, prepared by older salt fractionation methods, were analyzed in the ultracentrifuge. When purified, salt-fractionated immunoglobulin was subjected to the conditions of the Cohn fractionation process and subsequently analyzed in the ultracentrifuge the dimer peak was again observed. These experiments clearly demonstrate that ethanol fractionation induces dimerization of immunoglobulins. Nowadays it is known that these dimers are responsible for the anticomplement activity of ethanol-fractionated immunoglobulin; manufacturers of intravenous gammaglobulin who purify this fraction by the cold ethanol process therefore had to introduce additional steps to eliminate these aggregates.

Temperature

In the preceding paragraph we stated that ethanol denatures proteins, specially at higher temperatures, and that it causes aggregation of immunoglobulins. This does not seem to hold true for all proteins. In 1975 Schneider and collaborators (18) have proposed a new isolation scheme for albumin; according to their method, all plasma proteins except albumin are precipitated by heating plasma to 68°C for 30 minutes at pH 6.5 in the presence of 9% ethanol and 0.004 mol/L sodium caprylate. The pH is further lowered to 4.4 before filtration and further processing to a final product.

If this material is subjected to gel filtration on Sephadex G-200, a homogenous, symmetrical peak is obtained, which shows practically no trace of dimers or higher polymers (19); in contrast, albumin prepared by conventional cold-ethanol fractionation always contains about 2% dimers and 6% oligomers en polymers.

Human serum albumin contains one single cysteine group which is not involved in interchain disulfide bridges (20); in circulating albumin, some of these groups are involved in mixed disulfides (e.g., with half-glutathione). Therefore, when the number of free SH-groups in isolated albumin is assayed, a value below 1 is obtained. We found that albumin isolated by the cold-ethanol method contains 0.4 to 0.5 free cysteine group per albumin molecule; albumin isolated by polyelectrolyte adsorption (21) gave a similar value. However, albumin isolated by a heat-ethanol process contains only 0.05 free cysteine per albumin molecule (Morgenthaler, unpublished results). It appears therefore that heat-ethanol fractionated albumin is less aggregated than albumin isolated by the cold-ethanol method, but that the former is altered in some other way.

pH

The effect of extreme pH-values has been well studied in the case of albumin (reviewed in 20). Between pH 2 and 4, the molecule acquires an excess of positive charges, which force the protein into a more expanded form. This change in shape can be detected by measuring sedimentation, viscosity, and diffusion coefficients; the molecular weight of the protein is not affected. In an alkaline medium, albumin also undergoes isomerizations which are mediated by thiol-disulfide interchanges.

Acid expansion of albumin is reversible; since the changes in pH occuring to albumin during cold ethanol fractionation are less drastic it can safely be assumed that they inflict no permanent damage on this protein. Other plasma proteins, on the other hand, are less stable than albumin and can be damaged even by slight deviations from neutral conditions.

It has been shown several years ago that factor VIII activity is irreversibly lost when plasma pH was lowered from 7 to 4.9 (22); this has important implications for the collection on blood, since anticoagulant solutions (particularly ACD) can be quite acid. The authors estimated that 10 to 15% of the factor VIII activity are lost in the beginning of each donation, when the blood is mixed with excess anticoagulant. This deleterious effect can be avoided by continuously mixing the blood with the appropriate volume of anticoagulant.

Loss of cations

Many plasma proteins bind cations, the most important ones being calcium, magnesium, iron and zinc. Anticoagulation of blood is usually achieved by addition of chelating substances (e.g., citrate or ethylenediamine tetraacetic acid), by addition of precipitating agents (e.g., oxalic acid or fluoride), or by exchanging all other cations for sodium on an ion exchanger column. All methods used for anticoagulation therefore somehow interfere with the cations in the plasma and compete with the proteins for their binding.

It has been known for some time that calcium ions stabilize factor VIII; this finding has been reinvestigated recently and isolation methods for factor VIII have been proposed which avoid removal or complexing of calcium (references in 23). If blood is collected in heparin as an anticoagulant, factor VIII activity is more stable than when blood is collected into citrate solutions. If blood is first collected into citrate solution, increased stability can be observed after addition of heparin and calcium (fig. 1). Since the main difference between these various collection modes resides in the presencè or absence of free calcium ions, they are presumably responsible for the increased stability of factor VIII.

Shear forces

During fractionation, plasma proteins may be subjected to shear forces at various stages of the process. A large molecule like factor VIII would appear to be particularly susceptible to shear degradation. It is therefore interesting that concentration of factor VIII solutions by ultra-filtration could be achieved with almost 100% quantitative recovery (24). There are many places in the ultrafiltration apparatus (hollow fibers or flat membranes) and in the pump used for recirculation where high shear rates may occur. According to the authors, the liquid velocity had to be adjusted to maintain laminar flow throughout; the shear rate remained below 500/sec. The choice of a suitable pump was also important: air-operated diaphragm pumps performed far better than centrifugal pumps.

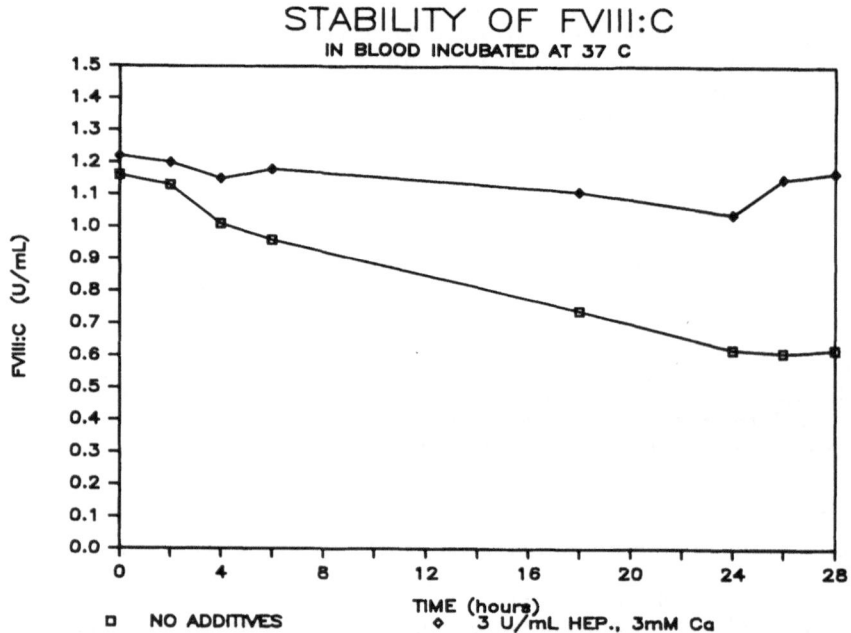

Figure 1. A blood donation was collected into ACD and divided into two aliquots; one was incubated without any other additives; to the other, 3 U/ml of heparin and 3mMoles/L of calcium chloride were immediately added. Both aliquots were incubated in parallel at 37°C; subsamples were taken at the times indicated and centrifuged. FVIII:C activity was measured in the supernatants with a one-stage assay.

Interaction with surfaces

It is now well established that most proteins bind to (plastic) surfaces; abundant use is made of this property in a variety of widely used assays. During blood collection and the fractionation process, plasma proteins come into contact with numerous surfaces: plastic bags, tubings, glass and stainless steel, and — last but not least — air.

Proteins can undergo structural changes when they adsorb on surfaces. This has been shown in the case of fibronectin, a large plasma protein (relative molecular mass 440,000) which is composed of several domains with distinct functions and binding sites. It has been shown that, at low concentrations, more plasma fibronectin is bound to hydrophobic than to hydrophilic surfaces. However, more antifibronectin is bound to fibronectin adsorbed on hydrophilic surfaces. Binding of antifibronectin to fibronectin adsorbed on hydrophobic surfaces increased in the presence of serum albumin (25). The conclusion from these experiments is that adsorption of fibronectin on surfaces depends on the nature of the surface and on the presence of other proteins in solution. Furthermore, both these parameters influence the conformation of the fibronectin molecule.

Enzymatic degradation

Plasma contains a whole range of proteases, either as active enzymes or as proenzymes (factors of the coagulation, complement, and kinin systems; plasminogen; trypsin). Their effect can be particularly detrimental on trace proteins (e.g., factor VIII). The biochemist has a whole arsenal of protease inhibitors at his disposal (soybean trypsin inhibitor; trasylol; heparin; benzamidine; epsilon-amino caproic acid; phenyl methyl sulfonyl fluoride; EDTA). Very few of these substances may be used in plasma fractionation, since they are either immunogenic or toxic.

Bacterial contamination

Human plasma is an excellent culture medium for bacteria. Bacterial growth destroys the proteins and adds endotoxins. Again, bacteriostatics and bactericids are available, but they may not be used in plasma fractionation, since they would contaminate the final product.

METHODS FOR DETECTING ALTERATIONS

Physicochemical methods

Although physicochemical methods are among the oldest tools for protein characterization, they are of limited value for assessing changes incurred during fractionation. As mentioned in the introduction, the problem of a suitable reference has to be solved first. Usually, the same protein is isolated by different methods and the properties of the various products are compared (26). As an extension of this approach, an isolated protein is refractionated by the same method and analyzed again; it might then be possible to detect cumulative changes. Finlayson has chromatographed albumin on DEAE cellulose; he was able to show that the elution pattern obtained changed with the storage time (thus with the polymer content) of the sample.

134

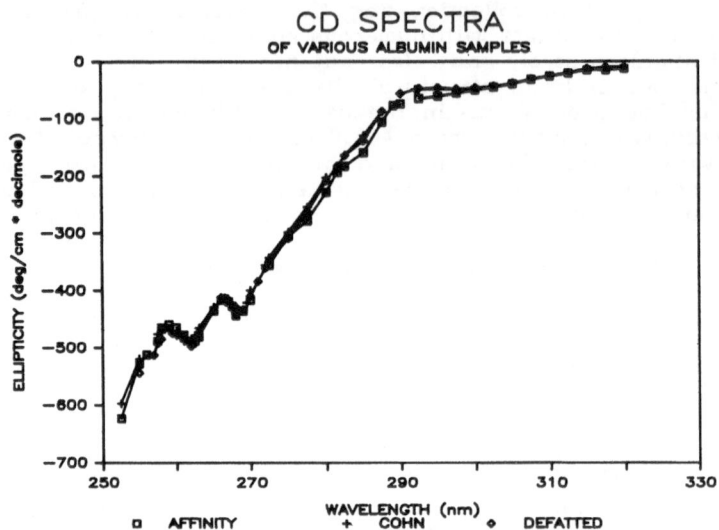

Figure 2. Affinity albumin was prepared by affinity chromatography on immobilized octylsuccinic acid; Cohn albumin is the routine cold-ethanol fractionated albumin of the SRC; the latter was also measured after being defatted with charcoal.

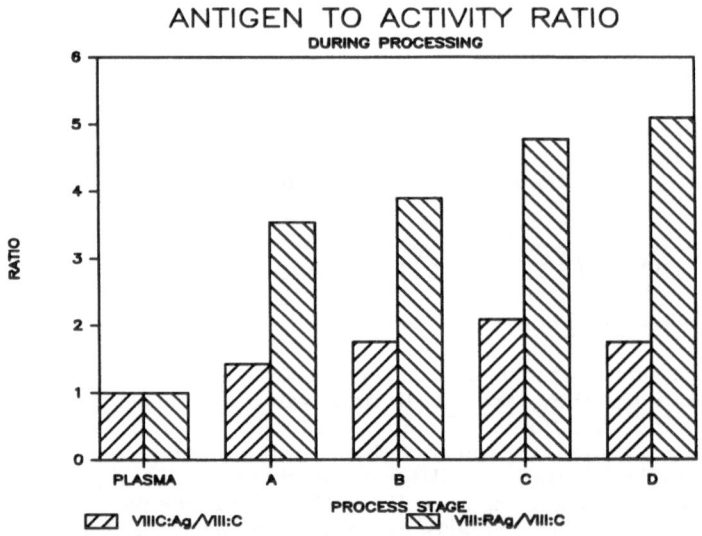

Figure 3. Process stages are: A: after tris extraction of the cryopreci-pitate; B: after aluminium hydroxide adsorption and citrate adjustment; C: after membrane filtration; D: after resolution of the freeze dried product. Ratios calculated from the data in (27).

We tried to detect differences between albumin samples prepared in different ways by measuring circular dichroism spectra. Fig. 2 shows 3 scans obtained with ethanol-fractionated albumin, ethanol-fractionated and subsequently defatted albumin, and albumin isolated by affinity chromatography on immobilized octylsuccinic acid. There are obviously no significant differences between the 3 tracings (Morgenthaler, unpublished results). This finding can be interpreted as a proof of structural similarity of all samples compared, or it could be the result of insufficient sensitivity of the method. Although parameters like diffusion coefficients, sedimentation constants, viscosity, CD/ORD spectra can give very precise answers for pure substances, they are difficult to interpret when a mixture with one dominant component is analyzed.

Biochemical methods

Biochemical methods are useful when the protein analyzed has a well defined activity. The activity per mass unit can then be compared in the unfractionated starting material and in the isolated product. This requires a precise measurement of the concentration of a particular protein in the starting mixture, which is usually done by immunological methods. In its natural surrounding, a plasma protein may self-aggregate, or bind to other proteins, thus masking certain antigenic determinants, or even exposing others due to conformational changes. Quantitation by immunological methods may therefore not be strictly comparable in different surroundings. We nevertheless use the ratio of factor VIII related antigen/factor VIII procoagulant activity as a quality criterion for AHF preparations. This ratio is 1.0 in the starting plasma, by definition. In commercial preparations, the ratio varies from about 2 to 10, which we interpret as an indication of partial denaturation of the factor VIII molecule: the higher this factor is, the more enzymatically inactive but still antigenically recognizable factor VIII is contained in a particular preparation. The increase of this ratio during the manufacturing process can be calculated from the values given by Prowse and collaborators (27) (fig. 3). Both factor VIII-related antigen/factor VIII coagulant activity and factor VIII coagulant antigen/factor VIII coagulant activity ratios are shown in this figure. The purification method used by the authors involves only extraction of the cryoprecipitate, adsorption with aluminium hydroxide, sterile filtration and lyophilization. Since no harsh treatment (e.g., precipitation) is imposed on the factor VIII molecule, the ratio goes up to moderate values only.

Enzymatic assays have to be interpreted with some caution. Thrombin has clotting as well as esterolytic activities. The enzyme can be made to loose both activities in parallel; certain treatments, however, destroy more than half the clotting activity, but leave the esterolytic activity practically intact. It is therefore important to measure an enzymatic activity against several substrates, and they should, whenever possible, include the natural substrate (26).

Denatured proteins are more rapidly digested by proteases; measurements of the rate of digestion therefore correlate with the conformation of a particular protein. Although the question of the appropriate standard still remains, it seems that increased sensitivity to proteases parallels a shortened intracellular half-life (26); in vitro degradation rate could therefore be another convenient method for assessing the potential damage a protein has suffered during fractionation.

Immunological methods

When an isolated protein is transfused back into a recipient of the same species, its immune system will recognize even small alterations in the organization of the molecule and help to eliminate it from the host's circulation. Turnover studies in a homologous system are basically very sensitive indicators of structural changes of proteins; however, a standard is again necessary, and the protein has to be tagged in some way. Although gentle methods for, e.g., radioactive labelling have been described, the protein will necessarily be altered, and this may affect the rate of its elimination. Animal proteins can be marked directly by incorporation of radioactive amino acids; for obvious reasons, this method cannot be used with human proteins. Experiments with ex vivo radioactively labelled proteins in humans have to be restricted also to a minimum.

The situation is altogether different when patients who lack a particular plasma protein are available. The half-life of factor VIII is normally measured in non-substituted hemophiliacs; survival of highly purified preparations can be compared with the behavior of un-fractionated factor VIII in plasma or in cryoprecipitate. Similarly, the half-life of isolated gamma-globulin can be measured in agamma-globulinemic patients (28).

Human proteins can easily be quantitated in the circulation of another mammal; the remaining concentration of, e.g., human albumin after injection of (unfractionated!) human plasma into a rabbit can be followed over the course of several days. Similarly, the disappearance of isolated human albumin after injection into another rabbit can be measured. The elimination rates of native (unfractionated) albumin and albumin isolated from fresh plasma were indistinguishable; therefore, purified albumin presumably keeps its native conformation. Isolated albumin which was reworked and contained high amounts of dimers and higher oligomers was eliminated at a faster rate. This heterologous system seems to be quite sensitive (26). Other authors confirmed and extended these findings (Tab. 1); reprocessed, but also heat-ethanol isolated albumin and purposely chemically altered albumin samples had significantly shortened half-life times (29; influence of chemical modification on turnover of proteins reviewed in 30). In the same study, new antigens could only be demonstrated on chemically modified albumin, but on none of the other albumin preparations tested.

Table 1. Half-life of various albumin preparations in rabbits

Albumin preparation	average half life (hours ± SEM)
Unfractionated albumin	143.0 ± 5.15
Pasteurized, cold-ethanol fractionated albumin	139.0 ± 14.75
Reprocessed albumin	125.1 ± 5.07
Heat-ethanol fractionated albumin	124.1 ± 5.25
Chemically modified albumin	79.9 ± 4.08

From (29)

CONCLUSIONS

Inspite of the far-reaching medical and commercial implications of this question, relatively little is known about the changes plasma proteins may suffer during fractionation. Although many different chemical and immunological methods are available, their application is usually hampered by the lack of a suitable standard. The best currently available evidence for the safety and efficacy of ethanol-fractionated human plasma proteins is their long-standing clinical record.

REFERENCES

1. Rothstein F. Some principles of plasma protein fractionation. In: Antoniades HN, ed. Hormones in human blood. Cambridge, Mass., Harvard University Press, 1976:3-31.
2. Kistler P, Friedli H. Ethanol Precipitation. In: Curling JM, ed. Methods of plasma protein fractionation. New York, Academic Press, 1980:3-15.
3. Polson A, Ruiz-Bravo C. Fractionation of plasma with polythylene glycol. Vox Sang 1972;23:107-18.
4. Farrugia A, Griffin B, Pepper D, Prowse C. Studies on the procurement of coagulation factor VIII: selective precipitation of factor VIII with hydrophilic polymers. Thromb Haemost 1984;51: 338-42.
5. Hao YL, Ingham KC, Wickerhauser M. Fractional precipitation of proteins with polyethylene glycol. In: Curling JM, ed. Methods of plasma protein fractionation. New York, Academic Press, 1980:57-74.
6. Newman J, Johnson AJ, Karpatkin MH, Puszkin S. Methods for the production of clinically effective intermediate- and high-purity factor VIII concentrates. Br J Haematol 1971;21:1-20.
7. Johnson AJ, Karpatkin MH, Newman J. Clinical investigation of intermediate- and high-purity antihaemophilic factor (factor VIII) concentrates. Br J Haematol 1971;21:21-38.
8. Steinbuch M. Protein fractionation by ammonium sulphate, Rivanol and caprylic acid precipitation. In: Curling JM, ed. Methods of plasma protein fractionation. New York, Academic Press, 1980:33-56.
9. Friedli H, Kistler P. Removal of ethanol and salt from albumin by gel filtration. In: Curling JM, ed. Methods of plasma protein fractionation. New York, Academic Press, 1980:203-10.
10. Curling JM. Albumin purification by ion exchange chromatography. In: Curling JM, ed. Methods of plasma protein fractionation. New York, Academic Press, 1980:77-91.
11. Falksveden LG, Lundblad G. Ion exchange and polyethylene glycol precipitation of immunoglobulin G. In: Curling JM, ed. Methods of plasma protein fractionation. New York, Academic Press, 1980:93-105.
12. Suomela H. An ion exchange method for immunoglobulin G production. In: Curling JM, ed. Methods of plasma protein fractionation. New York, Academic Press, 1980:107-16.
13. Brummelhuis HGJ. Preparation of the prothrombin complex. In: Curling JM, ed. Methods of plasma protein fractionation. New York, Academic Press, 1980:117-28.
14. Engvall E, Ruoslahti E. Binding of soluble form of fibroblast surface protein, fibronectin, to collagen. Int J Cancer 1977;20:1-5.
15. Morgenthaler JJ, Baillod P, Friedli H. Isolation of fibronectin under mild conditions. Vox Sang 1984;47:41-6.

138

16. Friedli H, Fournier E, Volk T, Kistler P. Studies on new process procedures in plasma fractionation on an industrial scale. II. Experiments in concentrating dilute albumin solutions using hollow fiber ultrafiltration. Vox Sang 1976;31:283-8.
17. Schultze HE, Schönenberger M, Matheka HD. Zur Kenntnis der Gamma-Globuline und antitoxischen Immunglobuline. Behringwerke Mitt 1952;26:21-57.
18. Schneider W, Lefèvre H, Fiedler H, McCarty LJ. An alternative method of large scale plasma fractionation for the isolation of serum albumin. Blut 1975;30:121-34.
19. Schneider W, Wolter D, McCarty LJ. Alternatives for plasma fractionation. Vox Sang 1976;31:141-51.
20. Peters T Jr. Serum albumin. In: Putnam FW, ed. The plasma proteins, vol. I. New York, Academic Press, 1975:133-81.
21. Johnson AJ, MacDonald VE, Semar M, et al. Preparation of the major plasma fractions by solid-phase polyelectrolytes. J Lab Clin Med 1978;92:194-210.
22. Vermeer C, Soute BAM, Ates G, Hellings JA, Brummelhuis HGJ. Contributions to the optimal use of human blood. VII. Stability of blood coagulation factor VIII during collection and storage of whole blood and plasma. Vox Sang 1976;31(Suppl):55-67.
23. Morgenthaler JJ, Zuber T, Friedli H. Influence of heparin and calcium chloride on assay, stability, and recovery of factor VIII. Vox Sang 1984;48:8-17.
24. Mitra G, Lundblad JL. Studies on ultrafiltration of antihemophilic factor. Vox Sang 1981;40:109-14.
25. Grinell F, Feld MK. Fibronectin adsorption on hydrophilic and hydrophobic surfaces detected by antibody binding and analyzed during cell adhesion in serum-containing medium. J Biol Chem 1982;257:4888-93.
26. Finlayson JS. Assessment of changes that occur in proteins during fractionation. In: Sandberg HE, ed. Proceedings of the international workshop on technology for protein separation and improvement of blood plasma fractionation. Reston, VA, Sept. 7-9, 1977:542-55 (DHEW publication No. (NIH) 78-1422).
27. Prowse CV, Griffin B, Pepper DS, et al. Changes in factor VIII complex activities during the production of a clinical intermediate purity factor VIII concentrate. Thromb Haemost 1981;46:597-601.
28. Morell A, Schürch B, Ryser D, Hofer F, Skvaril F, Barandun S. In vivo behavior of gamma globulin preparations. Vox Sang 1980;38:272-83.
29. Anhorn C, Sheldon S, Laschinger C, Naylor DH. Catabolic half-lives and antigenic relationship of native, altered and commercially prepared human albumins in rabbits. Vox Sang 1982;42:233-42.
30. Morgenthaler JJ, Nydegger UE. Synthesis, distribution and catabolism of human plasma proteins in plasma exchange. Int J Artif Organs 1984;7:27-34.

THE IMPACT OF DONOR SELECTION ON VIRUS TRANSMISSION

S. Iwarson

Transmission of different viruses via transfusion of blood or blood products is a well known problem and the virus mainly concerned today are the hepatitis non-A non-B virus(es) and the human T-cell lymphotropic retrovirus (HTLV/LAV) but also hepatitis B virus and some members of the herpes virus group will be discussed here.

Clearly, selection of blood donors in order to avoid certain well-defined groups at risk of transmitting AIDS or viral hepatitis have high priority world-wide. Besides these selection procedures screening for transmissible viral agents in the blood of potential donors is of great value.

The adoption of an all-volunteer donor system and the introduction of tests for hepatitis B surface antigen (HBsAg) effected a greater than 85 percent reduction in posttransfusion hepatitis (PTH). The incidence of PTH being 5-10 percent at most centres varying with the source of blood and transfusion volume. Of these residual cases, greater than 90 percent are due to the non-A non-B hepatitis (NANBH).

NON-A NON-B HEPATITIS VIRUS(ES)

There are many reasons to consider the non-A non-B virus(es) as one of the targets to concentrate on today. ALT-screening, which is far from ideal for NANBH-screening, has been introduced in a number of blood centres after some multicenter studies were presented. In two major american studies (Aach et al 1981, Alter et al 1981) ALT-testing appeared to identify a proportion of NANBH virus carriers among donors. Theoretical calculations indicated that screening of donors and rejecting of those who had ALT-levels above 45 units (normal less than 40 units) could precent 20-30 percent of PTH cases with loss of only 2-3 percent of the donor polulation. However, these were retrospective predictions based on the assumption that the donor with elevated ALT was the one to transmit hepatitis. In a later prospective study at NIH, in which all elevated ALT-units were excluded, there was no demonstrable reduction of posttransfusion NANBH (3). In addition, 60 percent or more of donor exclusions because of raised ALT-levels would be for non-viral causes, in particular obesity and alcoholism. Obviously the efficacy of both ALT and anti-HBc testing need to be assessed by further prospective, controlled trials before these test methods can be used as routine screening methods.

A recent discovery reveals that NANBH patients have the enzyme reversed transcriptase (RT) in serum. In this study, particle-associated reverse transcriptase activity was detected in four human serum specimens and in two plasma-derived products, all of which had been shown to transmit non-A non-B hepatitis to other humans and/or chimpanzees. Reverse transcriptase activity was also detected in all 12 sera from patients with acute or chronic NANBH. In contrast, reverse transcriptase activity was found in only 2 of 49 serum specimens from healthy plasma donors and laboratory workers. Sucrose density gradient fractions of two of the infectious human sera transmitted NANBH to chimpanzees. These data strongly suggest a retrovirus as one of or the only etiological agent associated with NANBH. This discovery will probably lead to a subsequent identification and characterization of the agent(s) causing NANBH and to the development of a test method.

General screening for reverse transcriptase in blood donors will probably not be possible because of the time consuming test method required and the costs, but in selected cases like donors implicated in NANBH among recipients reverse transcriptase analyses may be useful as a diagnostic test or a test of infectivity.

AIDS AND HTLV III

The AIDS problem and the possibility of transfusing the retrovirus HTLV III via blood or factor concentrates scares many recipients. In the USA about 50 cases of AIDS have been associated with blood trans- fusions and approximately another 50 AIDS cases have been noted in hemophiliacs. About 3 million individuals receive transfusions annually and about 20.000 US hemophiliacs are treated with factor concentrates. Why is the number of AIDS-cases in these large groups so far limited? Today studies are under way in the USA to find out the prevalence of antibodies to HTLV III among blood donors and the value of avoiding antibody positive blood. It should be remembered, however, that the number of tests required to be performed in the USA only in a general screening procedure is close to 25 million.

In discussing donor selection and screening an important point appears to be the improvement of blood bank effectiveness in terms of increased use of computerized information systems and operation research models. The AIDS problem has caused serious concern and educational programs have been instituted to inform persons at risk for developing AIDS to avoid blood donation as well as to inform personnel responsible for donor screening about AIDS. Since the victims of AIDS are also at risk for spread of for instance viral hepatitis, these programs may prove beneficial in reducing the transmission of viral hepatitis as well.

CYTOMEGALOVIRUS (CMV)

Cytomegalovirus, a member of the herpes virus family, is capable of causing latent infection and it is often difficult to distinguish a primary CMV infection from reactivation of a latent infection. Asymptomatic CMV infections frequently follow blood transfusions and the rare symptomatic infections are as a rule manifested as a heterophil-negative mononucleosis syndrome. In severely immunocompromised patients, CMV infection may result in more significant disease including persistent fever, pneumonia, hepatitis, pericarditis and encephalitis.

There is evidence that CMV seronegative blood products do not transmit CMV and hence that transfusion-associated CMV can be prevented. Infectivity is also thought to be reduced in leukocyte- depleted products including washed, frozen deglycerolized red blood cells and other leukocyte poor products. While CMV infections can be prevented by the use of seronegative donor blood, more specific markers of infectious blood would facilitate the provision of low infectivity blood products. While current serologic screening methods, including IHA, IFA and ELISA, have the necessary sensitivity to identify blood of low infectivity, they lack the desired specificity as shown by the fact that many seropositive donors do not transmit CMV.

Although donor screening and blood product manipulation do prevent transmission by blood to selected groups of severely immunoincompetent patients, such control measures are unnecessary for a very large majority of transfusion recipients.

EPSTEIN-BARR VIRUS (EBV)

Primary EBV infections occasionally may appear as the mononucleosis syndrome but usually remain silent. In either case, a latent viral carrier state ensues. Over 95 percent of adult blood donors have antibodies to EBV and are carriers of the virus. Therefore, EBV-bearing cells are transmitted daily by blood transfusions to thousands of recipients without causing disease. The percentage of susceptible recipients or blood decreases from its peak in infancy to approximately five percent in young adults and about one percent in old age. The majority of blood units transfused to susceptible patients are from viral carriers but besides EBV-genome carrying B-cells the blood contains EBV-neutralizing anti-bodies. Furthermore, the viability and functional integrity of lymphocytes are unimpaired in fresh blood but decrease gradually in the course of storage prior to transfusion.

It is logic therefore that symptomatic EBV infection follows blood transfusion only whèn the blood has been stored for a short period or time of the recipient has a T-cell deficiency of dysfunction.

These various considerations explain the rarity of EBV-induced mononucleosis following transfusion of blood and blood products and indicate that screening for EBV-markers as a rule is unnecessary.

HEPATITIS B VIRUS

Screening procedures for the detection of hepatitis B virus (HBV) using highly sensitive test methods for HBsAg have been introduced world-wide but one remaining problem is the occurence of so called "low-level" HBV carriers who are HBsAg-negative by routine RIA-testing but still infectious. Some of these "low-level" carriers may become positive when the serum sample is retested after for instance pepsin digestion. A simple and reproducible technique for the detection of these low-level HBV carriers would be of great value. A certain number of HBV-infected individuals have anti-HBc as the only serum marker of this infection. One question is whether transfusion-associated cases of hepatitis B could be prevented by testing all donors for anti-HBc and rejecting those positive. In fact the american "Transfusion-Transmitted Viruses" (TTV) study (1) tells us that anti-HBc screening of donors may reduce not only type B but also NANB hepatitis in recipients. In this study it was calculated that about 50 percent of the HB cases and about 12 percent of the NANBH cases could have been prevented through anti-HBc screening with loss of only about three percent of the donor population.

Well then, why do not all blood banks and plasmapheresis centres start testing for anti-HBc? One reason is that these calculations are theoretical and have not been confirmed in prospective studies. Another reason is that at least in hemophiliacs the impact of HBV will decrease rapidly in the near future when newly diagnosed cases can be vaccinated against the disease before receiving commercial or other clotting factor concentrates. Older hemophiliacs are as a rule immune to HBV infection.

REFERENCES

1. Aach RD, Szmuness W, Mosley JW et al Serum alanine aminotransfer-
   ase of donors in relation to the risk of non-A, non-B hepatitis in
   recipients: The transfusion-transmitted viruses study. New Engl J
   Med. 1981;304:989-94.
2. Alter HJ, Purcell RH, Holland PV, Alling DW, Koziol DE. Donor
   transaminase and recipient hepatitis. Impact on blood transfusion
   service. AMA 1981;246:630-4.
3. Alter HJ. Personal communication. 1984.
4. Seto B, Coleman W, Iwarson S, Gerety RJ. Detection of reverse
   transcriptase activity in association with the non-A, non-B hepatitis
   agents. Lancet, 1984;ii:941-3.

PREVENTION OF TRANSMISSION OF VIRUS INFECTIONS BY BLOOD TRANSFUSIONS AND REMOVAL OF VIRUS INFECTIVITY FROM CLOTTING FACTOR CONCENTRATES

R.J. Gerety

INTRODUCTION

Virus infections are serious complications following blood transfusions or intravenous therapy with clotting factor concentrates. Hepatitis A virus (HAV) is rarely transmitted by blood and never by plasma derivatives. Hepatitis A is characterized by a short viremia which most often coincides with clinical illness. In addition neutralizing antibodies to HAV are present in all plasma pools from which clotting factor concentrates are manufactured (1). Chronic Hepatitis B and non-A non-B hepatitis commonly follow acute infections (5 to 10% for hepatitis B, more than 40% and perhaps close to 100% for non-A non-B hepatitis). Chronic infections with hepatitis B virus (HBV) are characterized by serum levels of infectious virus up to 10^8/ml (infectious units) while levels of infectious non-A non-B virus are generally in the range of 10^2/ml (2,3). Little has been published concerning levels of HTLV III in blood or plasma.

The risk of infection by HBV, the agent(s) of non-A non-B hepatitis or HTLV III following receipt of clotting factor concentrates results from asymptomatic, chronic infections in blood and plasma donors, the manufacture of clotting factor concentrates from very large pools of human plasma, and the absence during manufacturing of steps which might remove or inactivate viruses. If the screening of donors by whatever means does not identify persons with virus infections, the consequences for the recipient of whole blood are obvious. With respect to plasma-derived products, however, other options exist to remove virus infectivity; these are outlined below.

VIRUS REMOVAL

The distribution of HBsAg and of HBV in plasma-derived products confirms that HBV preferentially distributes to fractions from which clotting factor concentrates are prepared (4 and Shih and Gerety, unpublished data, 1982). Attempts to remove HBV from a clotting factor concentrate by solid-phase immunoadsorption employing anti-HBs bound to Sepharose 2B have been summarized elsewhere (5). Similarly, crystalline polyethylene glycol (M.W. 4000) has been added to a clotting factor concentrate (this method is not applicable to factor VIII concentrate (AHF) since under these conditions factor VIII will precipitate out of solution) and the HBsAg/HBV removed by centrifugation (this study is also summarized in (5)). Both studies showed that HBsAg and HBV could be removed by these procedures, that each was relatively mild with respect to effects on clotting factors, but that neither could assure the consistent absence of infectious HBV in clotting factor concentrates. More recently Einarrson (6) showed that hydrophobic interaction chromatography can efficiently remove HBsAg and HBV from plasma and from clotting factor concentrates. Whether this procedure can assure the consistent absence of infectious HBV in clotting factor concentrates remains to be proved.

This latter method deserves further study, however, not only to remove HBV but for removal of the NANBH agent(s) and HTLV III as well. Neither antibody-mediated nor physical removal of infectious non-A non-B hepatitis virus(es) or HTLV III has been described.

IMMUNOLOGICAL NEUTRALIZATION

In 1980 one report (7) described the neutralization by anti-HBs confirmed by chimpanzee inoculations of more than 1,000 infectious doses of HBV intentionally added to a clotting factor concentrate. The addition of anti-HBs either during or after the manufacture of clotting factor concentrates appears to be a rather practical approach to preventing hepatitis B transmission while having little or no effect on the biological activity of the clotting factors. Although the addition of immuno globulin to clotting factor concentrates would appear to be new and to necessitate studies to determine the effect in recipients of repeated exposures to globulin, this is not the case. The globulin content of AHF can under normal circumstances approach 7 to 10 percent (Aronson, personal communication, 1983); most often this globulin has demonstrable anti-HBs activity, as well.

VIRUS INACTIVATION

In early studies, neither β-propriolactone nor ultraviolet light alone was capable of inactivating HBV although ultraviolet light did lower or remove HBV infectivity when applied in amounts which altered plasma proteins (8). The combination of β-propiolactone plus ultraviolet light has been reported to inactivate HBV (9). This combination of treatments has been applied to commercial preparations of some plasma-derived products. Alteration, denaturation or inactivation of proteins and residual β-propiolactone in products are concerns that have to be addressed if this combination of treatments is routinely applied to clotting factor concentrates.

Lipid solvents like alcohol and chloroform have been shown to inactivate enveloped viruses. Since retroviruses are the current major problems in plasma-derived products (being the cause of both non-A non-B hepatitis and AIDS) and since these viruses are enveloped, this method of inactivation is worthy of study.

Plasma clotting factors cannot routinely withstand heating at levels capable of inactivating viruses. Several plasma-derived products including Albumin and Plasma Protein Fraction are routinely heated at 60°C for 10 hours since this treatment can be applied in the presence of stabilizers and not adversely affect the biological activity of these products. The stabilizers in this case are acetyl tryptophanate and/or caprylate. This treatment is based on early data documenting the inactivation of HBV in Albumin by this combination of time and temperature (10,11). More recently, studies have evaluated methods to stabilize clotting factors to heating at 60°C for 10 hours since this treatment has also been shown to inactivate the retrovirus responsible for non-A non-B hepatitis (12,13). Unfortunately, since HBV can be inactivated in Albumin (11) but not in whole serum (14) by heating at 60°C for 10 hours, information about inactivation by heat may have to come from separate studies of each plasma-derived product. The inactivation in plasma of the retrovirus responsible for non-A non-B hepatitis (12) suggests that the sensitivity to inactivation by heat of this retrovirus is greater than that of HBV. Anti-thrombin III (AT-III) in 0.5M sodium citrate has been shown to withstand heating at 60°C for

10 hours with as little as 18 percent loss of biological activity in a rabbit model (heparin has also been shown to stabilize AT-III). In one study, more than 1000 infectious doses of HBV added to AT-III stabilized in 0.5M sodium citrate and heated at 60°C for 10 hours, did not transmit hepatitis B (15). The inactivation of HBV by stabilized AHF in solution has also been accomplished (16). In this study, the AHF was stabilized by dissolution in a saccharose/glycine solution followed by heating at 60°C for 10 hours and subsequent dialysis. HBV added to the pooled cryoprecipitate prior to manufacture of the AHF was inactivated by this process.

Theoretically, heating of stabilized plasma derivatives would inactivate HBV as well as the retroviruses responsible for non-A non-B hepatitis and AIDS. Data are needed, however, to assure that neither HBV nor agents of non-A non-B, or HTLV III are themselves protected by the conditions used to stabilize the clotting factors. Currently virus inocula with titered infectivity as well as serologic tests to assure susceptibility of chimpanzees are available for HBV inactivation studies. Few inocula exist for use in studies to assess the inactivation of non-A non-B hepatitis agents and the chimpanzee is required to assess lack of infectivity. HTLV-III containing inocula exist as well as methods for evaluating their inactivation in cell culture systems or by demonstrating removal of reverse transcriptase activity (14).

CONCLUSIONS

Screening tests, necessary to prevent the transmission of virus infections are essential to assure the safety of blood transfusions. An excellent screening test for hepatitis B (HBsAg) is available but none exist to prevent the transmission to recipients of blood of the retroviruses responsible for either NANBH or AIDS.

For plasma-derived products, additional means are available to prevent the transmission of virus infections by high-risk materials while preserving their biological activity. Either heating in the "wet" (preferred at this time) or the "dry" state should prove effective at removing infectivity of members of the problem virus group (retroviruses) responsible for non-A non-B hepatitis and AIDS.

REFERENCES

1. Smallwood LA, Tabor E, Finlayson JS, Gerety RJ. Antibodies to Hepatitis A virus in immune serum globulin. Lancet, 1980;ii:482-3.
2. Baker LF, Maynard JE, Purcell RH, et al. Hepatitis B virus infection in chimpanzees: Titration of subtypes. J Infect Dis 1975;132:451-7.
3. Tabor E. Propagation of hepatitis viruses in vivo and in vitro: Viral Hepatitis: Second International Max von Pettenkofer Symposium, Overby LR, Deinhardt F, Deinhardt J, Dekker M, ed. New York 1983:57-9.
4. Trepo C, Hantz O, Jacquier MF, Nemoz G, Cappel R, Trepo D. Different fates of hepatitis B virus markers during plasma fractionation. Vox Sang 1978;35:142-8.
5. Gerety RJ, Eyster ME. Hepatitis among hemophiliacs. In: Gerety RJ ed. Non-A, Non-B Hepatitis. New York, Academic Press 1981:97-117.
6. Einarrson M. Studies on the hepatitis B virus. Isolation of hepatitis B surface antigen from human serum and removal of hepatitis B virus from blood products. Doctoral thesis; Uppsala University, KabiVitrum AB, 112 87 Stockholm, Sweden 1983.

7. Tabor E, Aronson DL, Gerety RJ. Removal of hepatitis-B-virus infectivity from factor IX complex by hepatitis-B-immune globulin. Lancet 1980;ii:68-70.
8. Murray R. Viral hepatitis Bull. N.Y. Acad. Med, 1985;31:341-58.
9. Prince AM, Stephan W, Brotman B, van den Ende MC. Evaluation of the effect of betapropiolactone/ultraviolet irradiation (BPL/UV) treatment of source plasma in hepatitis transmission by factor IX complex in chimpanzees. Thromb Haemost, 1980;44:138-42.
10. Gellis SS, Neefe JR, Stokes J, Strong LE, Janeway CA, Scatchard G. Chemical, clinical and immunological studies on the products of human plasma fractionation XXXVI. Inactivation of the virus of homologous serum hepatitis in solutions of normal human serum albumin by means of heat. J Clin Invest 1948;27:239-44.
11. Murray R, Diefenbach WCI. Effect of heat on the agent of homologous serum hepatitis. Proc. Soc. Exp. Biol. Med. 1953;84:230-1.
12. Tabor E, Gerety RJ. The chimpanzee animal model for non-A, non-B hepatitis: New application. In: Szmuness W, Alter HJ, Maynard JE, eds. Viral Hepatitis: 1981 International Symposium. Phila.: Franklin Institute Press, 1982:305-17.
13. Seto B, Coleman Jr. WG, Iwarson S, Gerety RJ. Detection of reverse transcriptase activity in association with the non-A, non-B hepatitis agent(s). Lancet 1984;ii:941-3.
14. Soulier JP, Blatix C, Courouce AM, Benamon D, Amouch P, Drouet J. Prevention of virus B hepatitis (SH hepatitis). A J Dis Child, 1972:429-34.
15. Tabor E, Murano G, Snoy P, Gerety RJ. Inactivation of hepatitis B virus by heat in antithrombin III stabilized with citrate. Thromb Res 1981;22:233-8.
16. Heimburger N, Schwinn H, Gratz P, Luben G, Kumpe G, Herchenhan B. Factor VIII-Konzentrat, hochgereinigt und in lösung erhitzt. Arzneimittelforsch 1981;31:619-22.

INACTIVATION OF HEPATITIS VIRUSES (B, NON-A/NON-B) AND RETROVIRUSES IN POOLED HUMAN PLASMA BY MEANS OF β-PROPIOLACTONE-AND UV-TREATMENT

W. Stephan*, H. Dichtelmüller*, R. Kotitschke*, A.M. Prince**, R.R. Friis***, H. Bauer***

Drugs obtained from human blood, such as coagulation factors and anti-body preparations, are manufactured from large pools of plasma; this leads to contamination with viruses from a very wide range of groups.

We have taken up again a method of sterilization of human plasma used and published by LoGrippo in 1956. The essential advance entailed in this method (fig. 1) consists in the combination of chemical (β-propio-lactone) (β-PL) and photochemical (ultraviolet) (UV) sterilization. It must be stressed that this "cold sterilization" is only highly effective in the said combination. The individual steps alone are not sufficiently effective for the sterilization of plasma under mild conditions, as has been demon-strated in studies on volunteers by Murray (2) and Barker (3). Unfor-tunately the wrong conclusions were drawn from the then disappointing results, so that the work had been discontinued before the β-PL/UV combination had been tested.

COLD STERILIZATION TECHNOLOGY (5°-37°C)

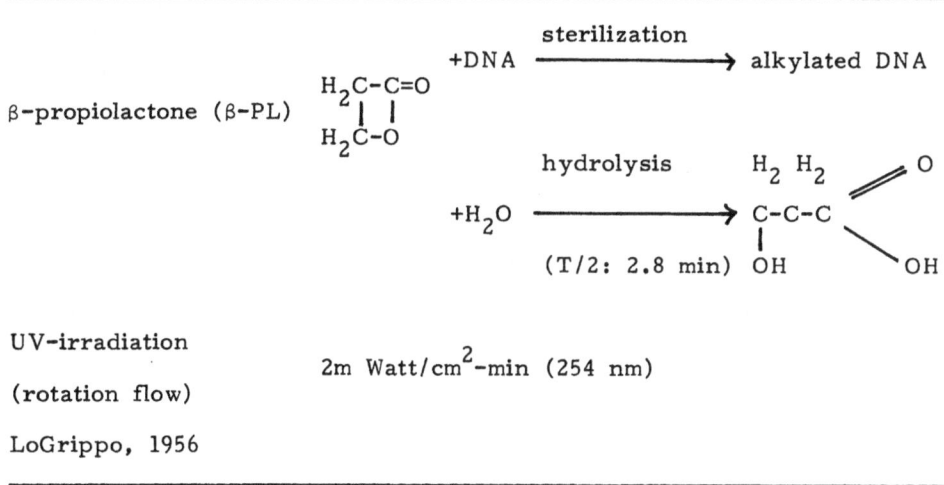

Figure 1.

*   Biotest Pharma, Frankfurt/Main, West Germany
**   The New York Blood Center, New York, N.Y., USA
***   Justus Liebig University, Giessen, West Germany

β-PL is a carcinogen but it decomposes very rapidly with a half-life of 2.8 min, in aqueous solutions and in the presence of plasma esterases. the β-hydroxypropionic acid formed by hydrolysis is not carcinogenic and is no more toxic than lactic acid. It is extracted from the reaction mixture by ultrafiltration of precipitation. together with other low-molecular substances. β-PL/UV-sterilized products have been tested by gas chromatography (4) and with the Ames mutagenicity test (5). As expected, no residual β-propiolactone or mutagenic activity could be detected.

Both β-PL and UV react with the nucleic acids of viruses, resulting in irreversible destruction of their genetic material. The UV irradiation is performed in a rotation flow apparatus developed in our laboratories, which allows the standardized irradiation of 1000 l-lots.

For inactivation of viruses in the presence of sensitive plasma proteins the main problem is to inactivate the viruses without destroying the plasma proteins. Yield losses have to be accepted, the latter varying from protein to protein (Tab. 1).

Table 1. Yield of plasma protein activity after β-PL/UV treatment of human plasma

Protein	Yield (%)	Parameters
Albumin	~100	Bilirubin binding
α_1-Antitrypsin	~100	inhibitor activity
IgG, IgM	~100	antibody activity
Fibrinogen	~ 90	coagulation activity
Factor VIII	~ 50	coagulation activity
PPSB	~ 50	coagulation activity

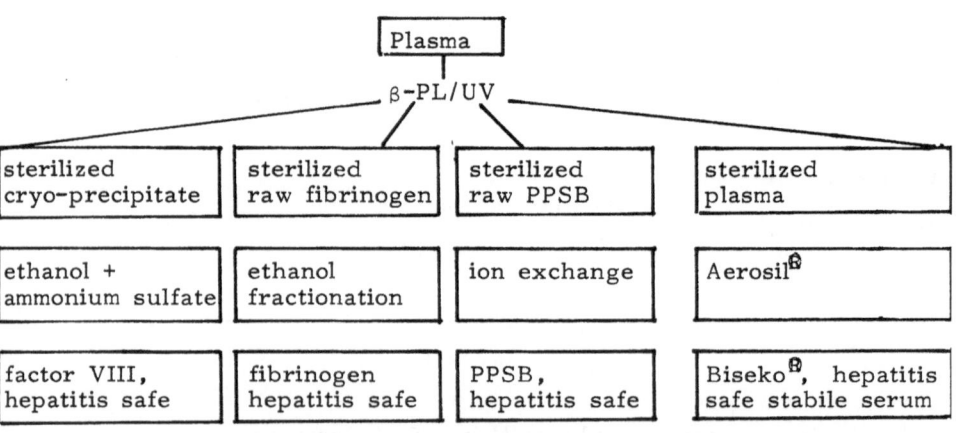

Figure 2. Fractionation of cold sterilized human plasma. Production scheme.

Table 1

Yield of plasma protein activity after
ß-PL/UV treatment of human plasma

Protein	Yield (%)	Parameters
Albumin	~ 100	Bilirubin binding
α_1-Antitrypsin	~ 100	inhibitor activity
IgG, IgM	~ 100	antibody activity
Fibrinogen	~ 90	coagulation activity
Factor VIII	~ 50	coagulation activity
PPSB	~ 50	coagulation activity

As can be seen, the serum proteins remain practically unaffected. Since the activities of the coagulation factors are reduced, special purification methods must be applied for their isolation. At Biotest this has resulted in the production scheme illustrated in figure 2. The cold-sterilized preserved serum Biseko[R] has been in clinical use since 1966 (6) and the PPSB concentrate since 1975 (7). Hepatitis safety has been demonstrated in chimp studies (,10), volunteer studies (11) and clinical trials (4,9). Factor VIII and fibrinogen are in the stage of scaling up. The in vitro en in vivo activity of experimental laboratory lots have been demonstrated.

The central step of Biotest fractionation process is sterilization with β-PL and UV. The key-studies and their results are summarized in table 2. More or less independent of the virus type β-PL/UV inactivates under standard conditions about 10^7 infectious doses/ml; the amount of hepatitis viruses which one can expect in screened plasma pools is between 10 (hepatitis NANB) and 1000 (hepatitis B) (A.M. Prince, personal communication). Thus β-PL/UV provides a considerable safety margin for production of safe products.

Table 2. Efficacy of β-PL/UV

Study	Inactivation
Stephan, Berthold 1981	$\sim 10^6$ CID_{50} HBV/ml
Prince, Stephan 1983	$\sim 10^7$ CID_{50} HBV/ml
Frösner, Stephan 1984	$\sim 10^8$ Hepatitis A-viruses/ml
Prince, Stephan 1983	$> 10^4$ CID_{50} Non-A, Non-B (Hutch. Strain)
amount of virus	$\sim 10^3$ HBV/ml
in screened plasma pools	~ 10 NANB/ml

The NANB study was carried out with hepatitis non-A non-B viruses in the form of the titered Hutchinson strain, the infectiousness of which is at least 10^6 CID_{50} (Chimpanzee Infectious Doses) per ml. This material was diluted 1:1000 with plasma of healthy plasmapheresis donors and treated with β-PL/UV under production conditions. Two chimpanzees were inoculated intravenously with 10 ml of the sterilized material. Neither animals developed non-A non-B hepatitis during a follow-up period of 203 days (fig. 3).

Transaminase levels remained within the normal range. Electron microscopic examination of liver biopsies, which were taken each month, revealed normal findings. Changes which are characteristic of a non-A non-B hepatitis could not be demonstrated in any case. The same animals were subsequently inoculated intravenously with 10 ml of the non-sterilized starting material — corresponding to an infectivity titer of at least 10^4 CID_{50} — in order to demonstrate both the infectiousness of the material used, and the susceptibility of the animals.

The results show that both animals develop definite non-A non-B hepatitis after this challenge. After approximately 30 days transaminase levels increased and the characteristic ultrastructural changes were seen by electronmicroscopic examination.

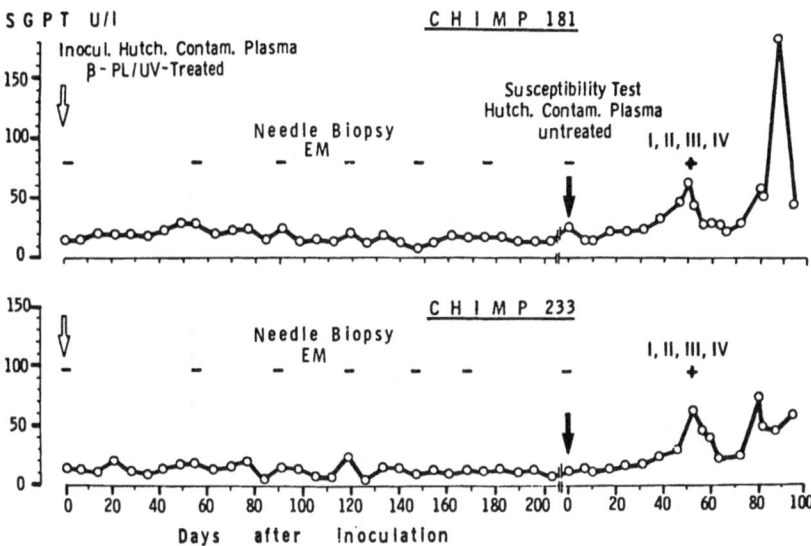

Figure 3. Results of follow-up of chimpanzees inoculated with 10ml of plasma contaminated with about $10^{3.5}$ CID_{50}/ml of Hutchinson strain NANB and then sterilized by β-PL/UV, and then challenged 30 weeks later with the same inoculum not subjected to this sterilization procedure.

Table 3. Inactivation of feline sarcoma virus (FeSV) and simian sarcoma virus (SiSV) by means of β-PL/UV

Sample	Foci/ml (mink cells)	FeSV Rev. transcriptase activity (cpm ^{3}H-Thymidin)	SiSV Rev. transcriptase activity (cpm ^{3}H-thymidin)
1000 ml Plasma + 10 ml FeSV (2.5×10^5/ml)	1 500	54 000	
1000 ml Plasma + 10 ml SiSV			22 000
–PL/UV treated plasma	0	4 200	1 700
Control	0	3 400	2 100
Infection Control	2 500	81 000	33 000

Inactivation of feline sarcoma virus (FeSV) and simian sarcoma virus (SiSV) by means of β-PL/UV

Sample	FeSV		SiSV
	Foci/ml (mink cells)	Rev. transcriptase activity (cpm ^{3}H-Thymidin)	Reverse transcriptase activity (cpm ^{3}H-Thymidin)
1000 ml Plasma + 10 ml FeSV (2.5 x 10^5/ml)	1 500	54 000	
1000 ml Plasma + 10 ml SiSV			22 000
ß-PL/UV treated Plasma	0	4 200	1 700
Control	0	3 400	2 100
Infection Control	2 500	81 000	33 000

Table 3

COLD STERILIZATION AND AIDS

Because the HTLV III virus from the group of labile retroviruses is discussed as a likely AIDS pathogen, we have treated human plasma contaminated with two animal retroviruses with β-PL/UV under standard conditions. Table 3 demonstrates that the combination of β-PL and UV is capable of inactivating retroviruses like the cat T-cell leukemia virus (FeSV) and the Simian sarcoma virus (SiSV). If the AIDS pathogen is indeed a retrovirus it should also be readily inactivated by β-PL/UV.

REFERENCES

1. LoGrippo GA, Hartman FW. Chemical and combined methods for plasma sterilization. Bibl. Haematologica 1958;7:255-30.
2. Murray R, Oliphant JW, Tripp JT et al. Effect of ultraviolet radiation on the infectivity of icterogenic plasma. JAMA 1955;157:8-14.
3. Barker LF, Murray R. Acquisition of hepatitis-associated antigen. Clinical features in young adults. JAMA 1971;216:1970-6.
4. Pruggmayer D, Stephan W. Gas chromatographic trace analysis of β-propriolactone in sterilized serum proteins. Vox Sang 1976;31:191-8.
5. Lissner RW, Pincus JH, Mortelmans K, Tanaka W. On the mutagenicity of β-propiolactone-treated therapeutic blood products. Lecture and Symposium Abstracts of the Hematology/Transfusion Congress Montreal 1980, No. 478.
6. Kornhuber B. Studie zur Hepatitissicherheit der Serumkonserve Biseko. Biotest-Mitteilungen 1974;35:44-5.
7. Köhler-Vajta K, Klose HJ, Frösner G. Klinische Prüfung auf Hepatitis-sicherheit eines "hepatitis-sicheren" Prothrombinkomplexes in pädiatrischem Krankengut. In: JR Kalden u. UD Koenig (Hrsg.) Blutkomponenten und Plasmaersatzmittel. Springer-Verlag Berlin, Heidelberg, New York 1982:113-6.
8. Prince AM, Stephan W, Brotman B. β-propiolactone/ultraviolet irradiation: a review of its effectiveness for inactivation of viruses in blood derivatives. Rev. Infect, Dis. 1983;5:92-107.
9. Heinrich D, Kotitschke R, Berthold H. Clinical evaluation of the hepatitis safety of a β-propiolactone/ultraviolet treated factor IX concentrate (PPSB). Thromb. Res. 1982;28:75-83.
10. Stephan W, Berthold H. Untersuchungen zur Hepatitissicherheit von sterilisierten Gerinnungsfaktoren aus Humanblut – Eine Schimpansenstudie. In: Kl. Schimpf (Hrsg.) Fibrinogen, Fibrin und Fibrinkleber. Nebenwirkungen der Therapie mit Gerinnungsfaktorenkonzentraten. F.K. Schattauer Verlag Stuttgart, New York 1980:321-5.
11. Prince AM, Stephan W, Brotman B. Inactivation of non-A, non-B virus infectivity by a β-propiolactone/ultraviolet irradiation treatment and Aerosil adsorption procedure used for preparation of a stabilized human serum. Vox Sang 1984;46:80-5.

HTLV-I/II AND HTLV-III SEROPREVALENCE IN BLOOD PRODUCT RECIPIENTS

T.L. Chorba, J.M. Jason, J.S. McDougal

INTRODUCTION

Human T-cell leukemia virus type I (HTLV-I) has been strongly im-plicated as the etiology of adult T-cell leukemia (ATL) (1-7), a T-cell type non-Hodgkin's lymphoma with leukemic manifestations in Japan, the Caribbean, and the southeastern United States (1-7). The prevalence of serum antibody specific for one core antigen of HTLV-I, p24, has been found to be high in patients with ATL (7-9), and higher in relatives of these patients than in general population controls (7-9). Reported population prevalences of p24 antibody have varied from less than 1% for U.S. and Japanese populations (7,8) to 3% for Caribbean populations (10). When antibody to another HTLV-I core antigen, p19, was evaluated, 0.5% of Washington D.C. participants, 1.9% of Georgia participants, 1.5% of Japanese participants from ATL non-endemic areas, and 11.9% of Japanese participants from ATL-endemic areas demonstrated antibodies to one of these core antigens (9). Recent findings suggest that HTLV-I is readily transmissible through cellular blood products (11,12), but not through lyophilized factor concentrates (13).

HTLV-II is a second subtype related to HTLV-I, with core proteins p19 and p24 immunogenically cross-reactive with HTLV-I. Although first obtained from a patient with a T-cell variant of hairy cell leukemia (14,15), HTLV-II has recently been isolated from a patient with a clinical presentation consistent with acquired immunodeficiency syndrome (AIDS) (16), and from a patient with severe hemophilia A (17). The mode of transmission of this agent remains unknown. Because of the immunogenic cross-reactivities of HTLV-I and -II, the presence of antibody to either of these agents is collectively referred to in this paper as reactivity to HTLV-I/II.

In 1983 it was reported that a significant percentage of hemophilia patients had serologic evidence of prior infection to HTLV-I or a related retrovirus (18). Whereas the HTLV-I, HTLV-II, and a new third sub-type, HTLV-III, have been isolated from T-cells of patients with AIDS (16,19,20,21), recent work has strongly implicated the cytopathic effect of HTLV-III on the OKT4-positive subset as the underlying pathogenesis of AIDS (22).

In order to assess the transmission of HTLV-I, HTLV-II and HTLV-III through blood components, we evaluated the anti-HTLV antibody status of recipients of cellular and non-cellular blood products and non-transfused healthy persons from New York City, an area of high incidence of AIDS.

METHODS

Participants

Participants were enrolled in 1983; details of patient selection and evalu-ation are given in detail elsewhere (23). Briefly, serum was obtained from 49 participants with hemophilia A who had received ≥100,000 units of factor VIII concentrate in the 12 years preceding their enrollment from two treatment centers in New York City. Only seven had received other blood products in the previous 5 years, for isolated bleeding incidents. These two centers treat approximately 40% of the patients with hemophilia in New York City. We also evaluated 48 persons with β-thalassemia major from a center that treats 67% of the transfusion-dependent patients with thalassemia in New York City; these persons had each received 12-24 units of frozen packed red blood cells per year in the previous 3 years, to maintain a hemoglobin level of >11mg/dl. Twenty-four patients with sickel cell anemia were enrolled from three centers in New York City that use routine transfusion therapy; these persons had each received ≥6 units of frozen packed red blood cells per year in the previous 3 years. Blood specimens were also obtained from 18 healthy New York City health-care personnel who volunteered to be controls for laboratory testing.

HTLV-I/II

The presence or absence of antibody to HTLV-I/II p24 and p19 was assessed by a sodium dodecyl sulfate/polyacrylamide gel electrophoresis (SDS-PAGE) and enzyme-linked immunoelectrotransfer blot (Western blot) technique described elsewhere (24), using HTLV-I purified from a T-cell line infected with HTLV-I (MT-2) (25). Details relevant to the present application are the following: SDS (final concentration 1%) and 2-mercaptoethanol (final concentration 5%) were added to purified MT-2 virus suspension. The preparation was heated at 65°C for 30 minutes and diluted 1:100 in sample buffer (1% SDS, 10% glycerol, 0,25mg/ml bromophenol blue, 0.01M Tris buffer (pH 8.0)). A 150-μl sample volume was electrophoresed on 3.3%-20% gradient acrylamide gels. PAGE-resolved proteins were electrophoretically transferred to nitrocellulose sheets, 60V x 3 hours, 4°C. The washed sheets were cut into strips and incubated overnight at 4°C with 1:100 dilutions of test serum. The strips were washed, incubated for 2 hours at room temperature with a peroxidase-conjugated anti-human Ig reagent, and washed again. Color reactions were developed with 3,3'-diaminobenzidine and H_2O_2 (24). Positive and negative sera as well as buffer control were included in all runs. Serum specimens were tested at a 1:100 dilution and banding patterns were compared with those of a known positive control serum.

HTLV-III

A similar Western blot analysis was performed using HTLV-III/lymphadenopathy (LAV) virus purified from HTLV-III/LAV-infected, phytohemagglutinin-stimulated human lymphocytes (26). Serologic reactions with any of the 18 kd, 25 kd and 41 kd proteins of HTLV-III/LAV were scored as positive.

RESULTS

All hemophilia A and non-transfused participants were negative for HTLV-I/II p24 antibody (table 1). Three (6%) of the β-thalassemia major patients and one (4%) of the sickle cell anemia patients were p24 antibody-positive. Three of these participants were also positive for antibodies to HTLV-I/II-associated p19 and p61 antigens; one β-thalassemia patient was positive for HTLV-I/II p24 antibody only. None of the

Table 1. Antibody status to HTLV-I/II-p24 core antigen by Western blot assay technique, by participant group.

Participant Groups	Positive Participants/ Total Tested
Hemophilia A	0/48
β-Thalassemia	3/48
Sickle cell anemia	1/24
Controls	0/18

HTLV-I/II p24 antibody-positive participants were born in the Caribbean nor had they traveled to Haiti, the West Indies, Japan, or Africa in the past 3 years. Information on blood product usage was obtained on 41 hemophilia A patients (median 419,500 units of factor VIII over the previous 3 years, range 16,470-1,444,260), 48 β-thalassemia patients and 22 sickle cell anemia patients. Blood-product usage by HTLV-I/II p24 antibody-positive participants ranged from a minimum of 26 units of frozen packed red cells to a maximum of 60 units of frozen packed red cells per year in the previous 3 years. Usage by HTLV-I/II p24 antibody-positive β-thalassemia patients was well within the range of the usage by the antibody-negative participants (median of 33-36 units per year in the previous 3 years). The antibody-positive sickle cell anemia patient had relatively high usage (median 35-60 units per year in the previous 3 years) compared with the antibody-negative patients (median 7-16 units per year in the previous 3 years).

Forty-four (92%) of the hemophilia patients had antibody to HTLV-III. Three β-thalassemia patients other than those who had demonstrated positivity for antibodies to HTLV-I/II had antibodies to HTLV-III. No sickle cell anemia patients had antibodies to HTLV-III. No controls were antibody-positive to HTLV-I/II or to HTLV-III.

DISCUSSION

The absence of antibody-positivity to HTLV-I/II in the hemophilia patients presented here treated with lyophilized factor concentrates is consistent with other data that indicate a lack of ready transmissibility of HTLV-I in such concentrates (17). The presence of antibody to HTLV-I/II in 1 sickle-cell anemia patient and in 3 β-thalassemia major patients, all of whom were chronically receiving frozen cellular blood product therapy, supports the hypothesis that HTLV-I is transmissible through cellular blood products and also suggests that freezing cellular blood products does not prevent HTLV-I transmission. Our data are consistent with the recent finding of increased prevalence of HTLV-I-antibody-positivity in frequently transfused sickle-cell anemia patients in Martinique (27). Insofar as HTLV-I is associated with ATL (1-7), transmission of this agent via blood products is a public health concern.

Although there is in vitro evidence that cell-free transmission of HTLV-I to non-lymphoid cell lines may be achievable under special conditions (28), most attempts to use cell-free HTLV-I-containing supernatants to infect normal human lymphoid cells have failed (29). These results would suggest that cell-to-cell contact is important for HTLV-I-transmission. This hypothesis has been supported by the finding of post-transfusion anti-HTLV-I-positivity in Japanese blood recipients who received cellular blood components from donors who where HTLV-I-antibody-positive, but not in those who received non-cellular blood components from HTLV-I-positive donors (30).

In contrast to the above findings concerning HTLV-I/II, our data showing that 44 (92%) of the hemophilia patients in this study had antibody to HTLV-III support the hypothesis that factor VIII concentrates may be a medium of HTLV-III transmission. Persons with hemophilia are at increased risk for AIDS, with 53 persons with hemophilia A and AIDS having been reported to the Centers for Disease Control (CDC) as of December 15, 1984. Ten of these had no record of having received any blood products other than factor concentrates in the 5 years preceding their AIDS diagnosis.

The differences in seroprevalence of HTLV-I/II and HTLV-III antibodies in hemophilia patients treated with factor concentrates and in cellular blood product recipients suggest these retroviruses have different modes of transmission or differing levels of infectivity in different blood components. Several considerations are important in interpreting these findings:

1. The sera assayed here for HTLV-I/II p24 may have contained other anti-HTLV-I/II antibodies that were not detected by these assay systems. It has been proposed that the absence of anti-HTLV-I p24 in some patients having antibody to the viral surface glycoproteins is likely to be a consequence of low immunogenicity of the HTLV-I p24 core protein rather than a lack of exposure to HTLV-I/II (30,31).
2. We may not have detected a low prevalence of antibody in persons with hemophilia because our sample size was inadequate. This possibility is unlikely in light of our similar findings in other hemophilia groups (13).
3. Factor concentrate is produced from donations made throughout the United States, while the majority of cellular blood products used by our participants came from donations made in the New York City metropolitan area. If prevalence of HTLV-I/II were higher in New York City blood donors than in those from other locations, these cellular blood products might be at higher risk of HTLV-I contamination than are factor concentrates, a reasonable possibility if persons at risk for AIDS are also at risk for acquiring HTLV-I (19,20,32-35).

These reasons might be given to explain an absence of antibody in our hemophilia population but do not discount the positive antibody findings in our β-thalassemia and sickle cell anemia groups.

The finding of evidence of antibody to HTLV-III in three β-thalassemia patients is of great interest because neither thalassemia nor sickle cell anemia patients are considered to be at heightened risk for AIDS; in none of the 44 transfusion-associated (non-hemophilia) AIDS cases reported to CDC as of February 8, 1984, had the patient received blood products for therapy of either of these hematologic disorders. Continued evaluation of these patient groups located in areas of high AIDS endemicity, and of the short- and long-term outcomes of HTLV-I/II and HTLV-III exposure is advisable.

In summary, the data presented here provide supportive evidence that HTLV-I/II is transmissible through cellular blood products and that HTLV-III is transmissible through factor concentrates.

REFERENCES

1. Blattner WA, Blayney DW, Robert-Guroff M, et al. Epidemiology of human T-cell leukemia/lymphoma virus. J Infect Dis 1983;147:406-16.
2. Akagi T, Ohtsuki Y, Takahashi K, et al. Detection of type C virus particles in short-term cultured adult T-cell leukemia cells. Lab Invest 1982;47:406-8.
3. Hinuma Y, Gotoh Y-I, Sugamura K, et al. A retrovirus associated with human adult T-cell leukemia: in vitro activation. Gann 1982; 73:341-4.
4. Gallo RC, Blattner WA, Reitz MS, et al. HTLV: the virus of adult T-cell leukaemia in Japan and elsewhere. Lancet 1982;i:683.
5. Blayney DW, Jaffe ES, Blattner WA, et al. The human T-cell leukemia/lymphoma virus associated with American adult T-cell leukemia/lymphoma. Blood 1983;62:401-5.
6. Popovic M, Sarin PS, Robert-Guroff M, et al. Isolation and transmission of human retrovirus (human T-cell leukemia virus). Science 1983;219:856-9.
7. Kalyanaraman VS, Sarngadharan MG, Bunn PA, et al. Antibodies in human sera reactive against an internal structural protein of human T-cell lymphoma virus. Nature 1981;294:271-3.
8. Kalyanaraman VS, Sarngadharan MG, Nakas Y, et al. Natural antibodies to the structural core protein (p24) of the human T-cell leukemia (lymphoma) retrovirus found in sera of leukemia patients in Japan. Proc Natl Acad Sci U.S.A. 1982;79:1653-7.
9. Robert-Guroff M, Kalynaraman VS, Blattner WA, et al. Evidence for human T-cell lymphoma-leukemia virus infection of family members of human T-cell leukemia lymphoma-virus positive T-cell leukemia-lymphoma patients. J Exp. Med 1983;157:248-58.
10. Schupbach J, Kalyanaraman VS, Sarngadharan MG, et al. Antibodies against three purified proteins of the human type C retrovirus, human T-cell leukemia-lymphoma virus, in adult T-cell leukemia-lymphoma patients and healthy blacks from the Caribbean. Cancer Res 1983;43:886-91.
11. Yamamoto H, Tometa N, Ishi A, et al. Blood products from anti-ATLA positive donors transform anti-ATLA-negative leukocytes in vitro. Cancer Res, in press.
12. Okochi K, Sato H, Hinuma Y. A retrospective study on transmission of adult T-cell leukemia virus by blood transfusion: seroconversion in recipients. Vox Sang 1983;46:245-53.
13. Chorba T, Jason J, Ramsey R, et al. Serosurveys for evidence of exposure to human T-cell leukemia virus (HTLV-I) in European and American hemophilia patients treated with factor concentrates prepared from U.S. plasma sources and in hemophilia patients treated with factor concentrates prepared from U.S. plasma sources and in hemophilia patients with acquired immunodeficiency syndrome. Thromb Haemostas, in press.
14. Saxon A, Stevens RH, Golde DW. T-lymphocyte variant of hairy-cell leukemia. Ann Intern Med 1978;88:323-6.
15. Saxon A, Stevens RH, Quan SG, et al. Immunologic characterization of hairy-cell-leukemias in continuous culture. J. Immunol 1978;120: 777-82.

16. Hahn BH, Popovic M, Kalyanaraman VS, et al. Detection and characterization of an HTLV-II provirus in a patient with AIDS. In: Gottlien MS, Groopman JE, eds. Acquired immune deficiency syndrome. New York, Alan R. Liss, 1984;73-81.

17. Chorba T, Brynes R, Telfer M, et al. Characterization of T-lymphocytes infected by a novel isolate of human T-leukemia virus type II (HTLV-II). Blood 1984;5(suppl 1), 201a.

18. Evatt BL, Stein SF, Francis DP, et al. Antibodies to human T-cell leukaemia virus-associated membrane antigens in haemophiliacs: Evidence for infection before 1980. Lancet 1983;ii:698-701.

19. Gallo RC, Sarin PS, Gelmann EP, et al. Isolation of human T-cell leukemia virus in acquired immunodeficiency syndrome (AIDS). Science 1983;220:865-7.

20. Miyoshi I, Kobayashi M, Yoshimoto S, et al. ATLV in Japanese patient with AIDS (Letter). Lancet 1983;ii:275.

21. Popovic M, Sarngadharan MG, Read E, et al. Detection, isolation, and continuous production of cytopathic retroviruses (HTLV-III) from patients with AIDS and pre-AIDS. Science 1984;224:487-500.

22. Klatzman D, Barre-Sinoussi F, Negeyre MT, et al. Selective tropism of lymphadenopathy-associated virus (LAV) for helper-inducer T lymphocytes. Science 1984;225:59-63.

23. Jason J, Hilgartner M, Holman RC, et al. Immune status of blood product recipients. JAMA, 1985;253:1140-5.

24. Tsang VCW, Peralta JM, Simons AR. The enzyme-linked immuno-electro-transfer blot techniques (EITB) for studying the specificities of antigens and antibodies separated by gel electrophoresis. Methods Enzymol 1983;92:377-91.

25. Kalyanaraman VS, Sarngadharan MG, Poiesz BJ, et al. Immunological properties of a type C retrovirus isolated from cultured human T-lymphoma cells and comparison to other mammalian retroviruses. J. Virol 1981;38:906-15.

26. Barre-Sinoussi F, Chermann JC, Rey F, et al. Isolation of a T-lymphotropic retrovirus from a patient at risk for acquired immunodeficiency (AIDS). Science 1983;220:868-71.

27. Fessain A, Gazzolo L, Yoyo M, et al. Sickle-cell anaemia patients from Martinique have an increased prevalence of HTLV-I antibodies. Lancet 1984;i:1155-6.

28. Clapham P, Nagy K, Cheingsong-Popov R, et al. Productive infection and cell-free transmission of human T-cell leukemia virus in an non-lympoid cell line. Science 1983;222:1125-7.

29. Miyoshi I, Taguchi H, Kubonishi I, et al. Type C virus-producing cell lines derived from adult T-cell leukemia. In: Hanaoka M, Takatsuki K, Shimoyama M, eds. Adult T-cell leukemia and related diseases. New York, Plenum Press, 1982;219-28.

30. Yamamoto N, Schneider J, Koyanagi Y, et al. Adult T-cell leukemia (ATL) virus-specific antibodies in ATL patients and healthy virus carriers. Int J Cancer 1983;32:281-7.

31. Lee CA, Kernoff PBA, Bofill M, et al. HTLV and hemophilia. Lancet 1984;i:1028.

32. Gelmann EP, Popovic M, Blayney D, et al. Proviral DNA of a retrovirus, human T-cell leukemia virus, in two patients with AIDS. Science 1983;220:862-5.

33. Essex M, McLane MF, Lee TH, et al. Antibodies to cell membrane antigens associated with human T-cell leukemia virus in patients with AIDS. Science 1983;220:860-2.

34. Essex M, McLane MF, Lee TH, et al. Antibodies to human T-cell leukemia virus membrane antigens (HTLV-MA) in hemophiliacs. Science 1983;221:1061-4.
35. Black PH, Levy EM. The human T-cell leukemia virus and AIDS. N Engl J Med 1983;309:856.

SERO-EPIDEMIOLOGY OF THE HUMAN T-LYMPHOTROPIC RETRO-VIRUSES HTLV-I AND HTLV-III IN THE NETHERLANDS:
Assessment of the risk of iatrogenic transmission by blood and blood products

J. Goudsmit

INTRODUCTION

The family of retroviridae encompasses all viruses containing an RNA genome and an RNA-dependent DNA polymerase (reverse transcriptase) enzymic activity. Only three years ago the first human retroviruses have been identified. Human T-cell leukemia virus (HTLV-I), the causative agent of adult T-cell leukemia-lymphoma (ATLL), has a type C morphology by electron microscopy, immortalizes T-cells in vitro resulting in continuous cell lines and is strongly cell associated (Table 1). A new human T lymphotropic retrovirus designated lymphadenopathy-associated virus (LAV) or human T lymphotropic retrovirus type III (HTLV-III) has been isolated initially from European patients with AIDS or at risk for AIDS and subsequently from large numbers of American patient with AIDS and at risk for AIDS as well. HTLV-III has a type D morphology by EM, is lytic to T-cells in vitro and is infectious in culture supernatants (Table 1).
    In the present paper the role of HTLV-I and HTLV-III in the etiology of ATLL and AIDS with the emphasis on the Netherlands is discussed. In addition the transmissibility of these viruses by blood and blood products is evaluated.

Table 1 Characteristics of T-lymphotropic retroviruses in humans.

HTLV-I	HTLV-III
C type by EM	D type by EM
Transforms OKT4 cells	lytic for OKT4 cells
Mg^{++} dependent RT	Mg^{++} dependent RT
Major core protein p24 unrelated to HTLV-III	major core protein p24
Major env protein gp46 related to HTLV-III	major env protein gp41
Stability in env gene	hypervariability in env gene
Strongly cell associated	infectious cell-free virus
Anti-HTVL-I neutralize	anti-HTLV-III do not

SEROEPIDEMIOLOGY OF HTLV-I IN THE NETHERLANDS:
THE ASSOCIATIONS WITH ATLL AND AIDS

The geographic and familial clustering of HTLV-I infection with ATLL strongly suggest that HTLV-I is the causative agent of adult T-cell leukemia-lymphoma (1-3).

Two main geographic clusters of ATLL have been identified, one in the Caribbean basin (2) and another in Southern Japan (3).

In the Netherlands, three black HTLV-I seropositive ATLL patients originating from Surinam and Curaçao have been reported (4) and in one case antibodies to HTLV-I, accompanied by expression of HTLV-I in peripheral T-cells, have been demonstrated in healthy relatives from the ATLL patients (5). An HTLV-I antibody prevalence of 12% has been observed in healthy Surinam emigrants participating in a methadon maintenance program in Amsterdam (6). The characteristics of these Surinam emigrants to the Netherlands are summarized in Table 2. Sera of 26 control Dutch iv drugusers lacked such antibodies with the exception of one female living with a Surinam male (6).

Antibodies to HTLV-I were detected in proportions varying from 5-15% in patients with AIDS and lymphadenopathy syndrome (LAS) from the USA (7) and Europe (8) when assays were employed, like ELISA using purified HTLV-I as antigen (7) or competitive RIAs (8), detecting mainly core related proteins. No such antibodies were observed in healthy homosexuals, the main AIDS high risk group (7,8).

Similar results were obtained in the Netherlands employing an ELISA with lysed purified HTLV-I as antigen. One of the 9 AIDS patients and three of 23 LAS patients had ELISA antibodies to HTLV-I relative to none of the 87 healthy homosexuals tested (9).

Table 2 Characteristics of Surinam emigrants with and without antibodies to HTLV-I**

Characteristic	Anti-HTLV$^+$(12)	Anti-HTLV$^-$(86)*
Mean age	28.2(12)	26.4(62)
Sex	75%(12)	90%(60)
Born in Surinam	100%(12)	95%(57)
Years in Netherlands	6.7(10)	7.3(54)

* Number in parentheses indicates number of cases for which characteristic is known
** Table compiled from M. Robert-Guroff et al (1984), Leuk Res.8:501

These data indicate that HTLV-I circulates among ATLL patients and their relatives, emigrants to the Netherlands originating from the Caribbean basin and among Caucasian patients with AIDS and LAS, who are severily immuno suppressed (Table 3).

Table 3 Antibodies to HTLV-I in all and AIDS patients and in individuals at risk for ATLL or AIDS in The Netherlands

Subject	Number tested	Number positive (%)
ATLL	2	2(-)
Surinam emigrants*	98	12(12)
AIDS	9	1(11)
Lymphadenopathy	23	3(13)
Homosexual men	87	0(0)
Normal controls*	26	1(4)**

* compiled from M. Robert-Guroff et al. (1984) Leu. Res. 8:501
** female living with a Surinam male

TRANSMISSION OF HTLV-I BY BLOOD AND BLOOD PRODUCTS

Transmission of HTLV-I most likely depends on the transfer of viable cells carying HTLV-I, because cellfree infection by HTLV-I, both in vitro and in vivo appears to be rare.

Blood transmission of HTLV-I has recently been demonstrated in Japan by a study of Okochi and co-workers (10); 63% of recipients of whole blood, or blood components with cells from donors having antibodies to HTLV-I seroconverted. No seroconversion was observed in either 14 recipients of fresh frozen plasma from HTLV-I seropositive donors or 252 recipients of whole blood or bloodcomponents from HTLV-I sero-negative donors.

Three Dutch hemophiliacs of 95 tested had antibodies to HTLV-I as tested by ELISA using purified HTLV-I as antigen (11).

One patient received cryoprecipitate as regular therapy, but several blood transfusions were documented as well. The other two received concentrate. This low frequency of HTLV-I seropositivity among Dutch hemophiliacs without an association with either cryoprecipitate or concentrate suggests accidental transmission of HTLV-I with contaminated whole blood or packed cells frequently administered to hemophiliacs in case of bleeding. Iatrogenic transmission of ATLL in conjunction with HTLV-I has not been reported to date.

HTLV-III INFECTION AND AIDS IN THE NETHERLANDS

Since AIDS emerged in the Netherlands during the fall of 1981 (12), over fourty cases have occured among male homosexuals. Table 4 shows the prevalence of antibodies to HTLV-III in patients with AIDS and at risk for AIDS in the Netherlands as tested by a specific indirect immuno-fluorence assay (13,14). Larger patient series, however, have to be studied to determine if these prevalences are fair reflections of sero-positivity in the Netherlands and not due to patient selection. These data indicate, however, that HTLV-III is highly endemic among both symptomatic and asymptomatic homo-sexual males. Only a minority of HTLV-III infected individuals appear to develop AIDS indicating that antibodies to HTLV-III do not protect against progression of the disease.

Within the main AIDS-high risk group of homosexual males the prevalence of HTLV-III infection is remarkably higher than that of clinically manifest immunosuppresion indicating a variability of the host response to HTLV-III infection from subclinical to severe, like to cytomegalovirus or hepatitis B virus.

Table 4 Antibodies to HTLV-III in patients with AIDS and at risk for AIDS

Subject	Number tested	Number positive (%)
Aids	11	5(46)
Lymphadenopathy	13	8(62)
Homosexual men	15	5(33)
Hemophiliacs	18	5(28)
Normal controls	12	0(-)

TRANSMISSION OF HTLV-III AND AIDS BY BLOOD AND BLOOD PRODUCTS

AIDS is transmissible through transfusion of blood (15) and the administration of blood products, in particular to hemophiliacs (16). HTLV-III has been isolated from a hemophiliac AIDS case (17). HTLV-III has been recovered from a blood donor's peripheral lymphocytes 12 months after the onset of AIDS and from the blood recipient's lymphocytes 1 month after her onset of AIDS symptoms (17). An extremely high prevalence of antibodies to HTLV-III has been observed among American (18) and European asymptomatic hemophiliacs. In the Netherlands a similarly high prevalence (31%) of HTLV-III seropositivity has been observed in a small number of sera taken in 1983 from hemophiliacs. None of the 6 recipients of cryoprecipitate without documented administration of other blood products, 3 of 7 recipients of factor VIII concentrate with or without blood transfusion and none of three recipients of PCC without blood transfusions had antibodies to HTLV-III. Two HTLV-III seropositive hemophiliacs received besides cryoprecipitate or PCC also blood transfusions on several occasions. In the Netherlands no AIDS cases among hemophiliacs have been reported yet. The high prevalence of HTLV-III seropositivity among hemophiliacs receiving factor VIII concentrate has to be set against the low prevalence of AIDS in this risk group thusfar. It indicates the presence of HTLV-III or its antigens in pooled blood products. Because of the cell-free infectivity of HTLV-III in vitro, HTLV-III is more likely than HTLV-I to be transmitted from concentrates prepared from large donors pools, contaminated with virus.

PREVENTION OF T-LYMPHOTROPIC RETROVIRUS TRANSMISSION BY BLOOD AND BLOOD PRODUCTS

I. HTLV-I

HTLV-I has been shown to circulate in emigrants to the Netherlands originating from the Caribbean basin. Because seropositivity has been shown to correlate well with the presence of infectious HTLV-I in peripheral blood, assays specific for serum antibodies to HTLV-I can be used to predict circulating antigen. It has to be considered to exclude family members of ATLL patients from blood donation and to test donated blood of individuals originating from HTLV-I endemic areas for the presence of antibodies to HTLV-I. Because of the sometimes low specificity of first generation tests for antibodies to HTLV-I. ELISAs or RIAs for the specific detection of the major core protein of HTLV-I, p24 should be used for this goal if available.

II. HTLV-III

HTLV-III has been shown to circulate among Caucasian homosexual males in the Netherlands and possibly among intravenous drug users, like in England and emigrants from AIDS endemic regions, like central Africa and the Caribbean basin. Because of the rapid spred of HTLV-III infection in the homosexual community. the cell free infectivity of HTLV-III and the wide spread occurrence of AIDS among HTLV-III infected individuals, prevention of HTLV-III transmission by blood and blood products should be first priority. The following measures should be considered:
1. Individuals at risk for AIDS, i.c. homosexual males and i.v. drug abusers should be discouraged to donate blood.
2. All units of donor blood should be tested for HTLV-III antigen or antibodies to HTLV-III and excluded if positive. The first generation test (like IFA, RIA and ELISA using whole virus or virus infected cells as antigen)appear to be more specific for HTLV-III antibodies than similar tests for antibodies to HTLV-I and could be suitable for screening of blood. However, specificity of the individual tests still has to be tested and some seronegative individuals from AIDS risk groups have been shown to carry virus indicating the need for an antigen assay.
3. Hemophiliacs should be treated with cryoprecipitate or with (locally produced) concentrate prepared from HTLV-III seronegative donors.
4. HTLV-III can be readily inactivated (if in solution) by heating products to 56° C for 30 minutes or treatment with 25% ethanol, 1% glutaraldehyde or 0.2% sodium hypochlorite for at least 30 minutes. Blood products like gamma globulins, human blood derived vaccines or factor VIII preparations should be inactivated by a treatment known to inactive these viruses.

REFERENCES

1. Poiesz BJ, Ruscetti FW, Gazdar AF, et al. Detection and isolation of type C retrovirus particles from fresh and cultured lymphocytes of a patient with cutaneous T-cell lymphoma. Proc Natl Acad Sci 1980; 77:7415-9.
2. Catovsky C, Greaves MF, Rose M, et al. Adult T-cell lymphoma-leukemia in blacks from the West Indies. Lancet 1982;i:639-43.
3. Uchiyama T, Yodoi J, Sagawa K, et al. Adult T-cell leukemia in Japan: Clinical and hematologic features of 16 cases. Blood 1977; 50:481-92.
4. Miedema F. Terpstra FG, Smit JW, et al. Functional properties of neoplastic T-cells in adult T-cell lymphoma/leukemia patients from the Caribbean. Blood 1984;63:477-81.

5. Vyth-Dreese FA, Rümke P, Robert-Guroff M, et al. Antibodies against human T-cell leukemia/lymphoma virus (HTLV) and expression of HTLV p19 antigen in relatives of a T-cell leukemia patient originating from Surinam. Int J Cancer 1983;32:337-42.
6. Robert-Guroff M, Coutinho RA, Zadelhoff AW, et al. Prevalence of HTLV-specific antibodies in Surinam emigrants to the Netherlands. Leuk Res 1984;8:501-4.
7. Robert-Guroff M, Blayney DW, Safai B, et al. HTLV-I-specific antibody in AIDS patients and others at risk. Lancet 1984;ii:128-31.
8. Tedder R, Shanson D, Jeffries D, et al. Low prevalence in the UK of HTLV-I and HTLV-II infection in subjects with AIDS, with extended lymphadenopathy, and at risk of AIDS. Lancet 1984;ii: 125-8.
9. Goudsmit J, Miedema F, Wijngaarden-du Bois RJGJ, et al. Immunoglobulin subclasses of antibodies to HTLV-I associated antigens in AIDS and Lymphadenopathy Syndrome. J. Virol: in press.
10. Okochi K, Sato H, Hinuma Y. A retrospective study on transmission of adult T-cell leukemia virus by blood transfusion: seroconversion in recipients. Vox Sang 1983;46:245-53.
11. Goudsmit J, Miedema F, Breederveld C, et al. Antibodies to the human T-lymphotropic retrovirus HTLV-I in Dutch haemophiliacs. Vox Sang (submitted).
12. Goudsmit J, Wertheim-van Dillen P, Schellekens PThA, et al. Acquired Immune Deficiency Syndrome, altered T-cell subset ratios and cytomegalovirus infections among male homosexuals in the Netherlands. Antibiot Chemother. 1984;32:138-46.
13. Cheingsong-Popov R, Weiss RA, Dalgleish A, et al. Prevalence of antibody to human T-lymphotropic virus type III in AIDS and AIDS-risk patients in Britain. Lancet 1984;ii:477-80.
14. Goudsmit J, Tersmette T, Kabel P, et al. IgG antibodies to HTLV-III associated antigens in patients with AIDS and at risk for AIDS in the Netherlands. AIDS Res. (in press).
15. Andreani T, Modigliani Y, Le Charpentier A, et al. Acquired immunodeficiency with intestinal cryptosporidiosis: possible transmission by Haitian whole blood. Lancet 1983;i:1187-91.
16. Ragni MV, Lewis JH, Spero JA, et al. Acquired immunodeficiency-like syndrome in two haemophiliacs. Lancet 1983;i:213-4.
17. Feorino PM, Kalyanaraman VS, Haverkos HW, et al. Lymphadenopathy associated virus infection of blood donor − recipient pair with acquired immunodeficiency syndrome. Science 1984;225:69-72.
18. Ramsey RB, Palmer EL, McDougall EL, et al. Antibody to LAV in haemophiliacs with and without AIDS. Lancet 1984;ii:397-8.

DISCUSSION

Moderators: R.A. Coutinho H.H. Gunson

C.V. Prowse:

Dr. Nydegger, in your list in the beginning, you mentioned the possibility of using neo-antigen assays as a method of measuring denaturation. Have you any experience with that, and how sensitive do you think it is?

U.E. Nydegger (Bern):

We have indeed measured neo-antigenic determinants. We did not want to call these new antigens, because the issue of neo-antigens is more a qualitative appreciation assessed by crossreactivities than a possibility to quantitatively measure new antigens. The modification is very subtle. Thus, if you do a double diffusion test, you find total antigenic identity.

C.Th. Smit Sibinga:

Dr. Nydegger, you showed quite nicely that, during the conventional fractionation methodologies, specifically albumin and more evidently immunoglobulins are affected basically by the process of purification. Therefore, if you want to inject the IgG's intravenously, you have to do some further chemical processing to get rid of the polymers to eventually get a safe product which has the potency you wish it to have. Do you not think it is a better approach to start thinking of processes in which you do not have this initial change in the molecules and the polymerization, instead of fiddling around with other chemical processes to eventually obtain a safe product?

U.E. Nydegger:

That is a very good question, but I can cite here one of my teachers S. Barandun, who always says: "IgG molecules are like little children. If you leave them alone — in other words, if you purify them to 100% purity — then they tend to aggregate and form little groups". In anyone procedure you may use to purify IgG, the purer IgG will have a tendency to aggregate, because of the abundance of non-polar groups, the large hydrophobicity and the complicated tertiary structure of the molecule. So I do not think that the aggregation tendency of IgG can be influenced by any of the purification methods used. One has to treat the product so that it is finally devoid of aggregates.

In this connection, it is noteworthy that a very small content of aggregates does not harm normo-gammaglobulinemic patients. They are only a problem in hypo-gammaglobulinemics, so in humoral immunodeficiency patients, who are highly susceptible to the slightest amounts of aggregates in such preparations.

J.B. Bussel (New York):

Could you review what is known about heat-treating proteins? At least in the United States, there is a lot of concern about what the heat-treatment of FVIII concentrates might do to the FVIII molecule. But this treatment is also done for antithrombin III concentrates and other things. Is there any work on what this does?

U.E. Nydegger:

Dr. B. Horowitz, from the New York Blood Center, has presented data at the last ISBT Congress in Munich (1) that changes can be seen in gel electrophoresis and crossed immunoelectrophoresis after heating purified clotting factor VIII.

I.M. Nilsson (Malmø):

How did you measure VIII:C in the plasma to which you had added three units of heparin per ml and calcium?

U.E. Nydegger:

In this case, we did a one-stage assay.

I.M. Nilsson:

Did you neutralise the heparin?

U.E. Nydegger:

Heparin was adsorbed on Cellex T before the activity measurement.

E.L. Snyder (New Haven):

Dr. Iwarson, you showed the number of AIDS cases related to trans-fusion as 100; when divided into 3 million, you came up with a figure of one in 30,000. Those cases of around 100 should be divided over 15 million, because those 100 cases have been collected over five years, and were not the number of cases due to transfusion in one year. So, the number is really closer to 1 in 150,000 than in 30,000.

One other comment you made: You suggested that perhaps the test for hepatitis C — if I can use that term — should be reserved for people that are at higher risk. But considering what is going on in the United States with ALT testing and the HTLV-III test, I do not see how we can avoid using a test for hepatitis C — if one becomes available. The concern I have is, by what extent it is going to increase the cost of medical care. I know very little about the immunology of retroviruses.

1. Horowitz B, Prince AM, Wiebe ME. Inactivation of viruses in labile blood derivatives. In: Abstracts of the 18th Congress of the ISBT, S. Karger Basel, 1984:77.

Is it possible to have a test which could be able to identify retroviruses in general and then if those are positive, go on to subsequently identify what type it is and use that as a screening test? Otherwise, we are going to add millions of dollars to the cost of medical care every time another retrovirus is identified.

S. Iwarson (Götenborg):

So far only about 1% of the reported AIDS-cases is possibly associated with blood transfusion and the incidence of AIDS per unit transfused will be more or less a guess since too many uncertainties are involved in the calculations. This does not mean that I oppose to your suggestions concerning the possible incidence of AIDS following transfusions.

As regards your second comment, I just want to point out that we are still in an early phase of research for reverse transcriptase (RT) and non-A non-B hepatitis. I think we all agree with you that if serum-RT can be used as a screening test for retrovirus infections many things would be much easier.

R.A. Coutinho (Amsterdam):

May I add another question? Is there any evidence of cross reactivity between the non-A non-B virus and HTLV-I and HTLV-III?

R.J. Gerety (Bethesda):

I think there are some preliminary data. It is possible that an individual multiply exposed to non-A non-B hepatitis agents, could develop limited antibodies with cross-reactivity against HTLV-III. We have purified an antigen from non-A non-B hepatitis, a glycoprotein; if you hyperimmunise an animal with this material, you begin to get reactivity against HTLV-III. It is, of course, a reactivity to a single protein.

W.G. van Aken (Amsterdam):

My question is initiated by the presentation of Dr. Goudsmit and in fact related to the anti HTLV-III screening of blood donations. His rather provocative recommendation should be open for discussion, since at least I am not aware of very firm data about the sensitivity and the specificity of anti HTLV-III screening tests.

I think this is necessary before we can make recommendations to blood centres as to whether they should or should not yet apply tests in routine screening. We should all agree that these are far-ranging conclusions. What are we going to tell the donors? How are we going to exclude them? What sort of confirmatory tests do we have to perform? So, before we leave Groningen tonight, we all should be aware of these problems. We have a panel here what may be able to discuss this. I would like to ask what the members of the panel think of the recommendations which Dr. Goudsmit has presented.

R.A. Coutinho:

I think that the first and the most important question is: What do we know about the sensitivity and specificity of the tests which are going to be marketed in the next couple of months?

C.Th. Smit Sibinga:

I fully agree with Prof. van Aken. I have information which I brought from the AABB session on AIDS (2) which might contribute to this extremely important discussion. It was quite firmly stated at the AABB that this test is not a test for AIDS, it is a test on an antibody related to a retrovirus which has a certain relationship to AIDS, as we learned today.

Table. Anti-HTLV-III Serology

Sensitivity = 95%					Specificity = 99%	
Incidence/ 100,000	++ A	-+ B	+- C	-- D	PVP(%)	PVN(%)
2	1.9	1,010	0.1	98,987.9	0.19	99.99
4	3.8	1,010.1	0.2	98,985.9	0.38	99.99
20	19	1,009.9	1	98,970.1	1.84	99.99
40	38	1,009.7	2	98,950.3	3.62	99.99

The table shows the membrane associated antibody test to have a sensitivity of 95% and a specificity of 99%, and gives the incidence on a population of 100,000: Low incidence areas of 2 and 4, high incidence areas of 20 and 40 cases. The next four columns show the incidences on positivity and negativity of the test. Column A indicates the true positives. The second column B means no symptoms at all, no history, or apparently not belonging to any risk category. You could raise the question of what that actually means. The plus is a positive test, so that could be defined as a false positive.

The third and the fourth column refer to the false negatives and true negatives. Finally, the incidences of the false positives and the false negatives are given. The major worry which came up at the discussion, was over the second column, the munis-plus "false positives". What does it actually mean when we find a positive test in a donor not belonging to any risk group, not showing any symptoms, not having any history related to AIDS. What are we going to do with this kind of information.

J. Goudsmit (Amsterdam):

I wanted to know which tests we are talking about here. Is this the immunofluorescence?

C.Th. Smit Sibinga:

This is an ELISA confirmed in the Western blot method.

2. AIDS: An informative update. 37th Annual meeting AABB, San Antonio TX, 1984.

J. Goudsmit:

I think that there are a few important questions. The first one, considering the data is: What are false positives? For instance a fluorescence assay picks up mainly glycoproteins, expressed on the membrane of those cells, which as we know can crossreact with other virus glycoproteins. If there are a lot of retroviruses crossreacting, it could very well be that these are not false positives in the sense of fals positives for retroviruses in general; they are false positives for HTLV-III in particular. To make it more provocative, it may very well be that this is an advantage, because those are people with other retroviruses whom you have to exclude anyway. So perhaps those false positives are a lucky thing, in this situation.

C.Th. Smit Sibinga:

Do you mean that these false positives — this is another provocative statement — could be a cross-sensitivity to the non-A non-B or another retrovirus?

J. Goudsmit:

That could very well be. For screening, that kind of false positivity therefore maybe a lucky circumstance.

R.J. Gerety:

With respect to the HTLV-III antibody test, I can give you my view from the perspective of the United States only. In the U.S.A., we have declared the test for antibodies to HTLV-III to be a biological one. It will go through the same rigorous evaluation as did hepatitis B surface antigen tests. Clinical studies utilising such tests are being done currently by five manufacturers all of whom are using ELISA technology. Reactive samples will be repeat tested, they will be confirmed by Western blot or other method and they will be provided to the FDA for the assessment of particle-associated reverse transcriptase, cultures and the like.

A Department of Health and Human Services study involves the sera from 15,000 blood donors tested. For confirmation of the analysis repeat tests are done by the Western blot or other method, looking for particle associated reverse transcriptase and virus by culture. At the end of all these studies, we will be able to say whether or not antibody correlates with presence of viable virus as detected by reverse transcriptase containing particles and/or culture positivity. All biologicals licensed in the U.S.A., like the hepatitis B surface antigen tests, require a confirmatory test. I am not at liberty to talk about all the confirmatory tests that manufacturers are developing, but each of the five manufacturers will have a confirmatory test to confirm the presence of specific antibodies and perhaps even specific virus antigens, or specific viruses either at the time of or soon after license of the tests.

W.G. van Aken:

Could you give us an idea about when these studies will be finished?

R.J. Gerety:

Because of the numbers of plasma donors donating in the U.S.A. and the cooperation between the manufacturers and the plasma and blood industry, we are projecting that in two months we will have the clinical data available. The test will be a licensed biological in the U.S.A. and a required one.

W.G. van Aken:

Dr. Gerety, in view of your preliminary data showing that there may exist crossreactivity between non-A non-B and HTLV-III, how is that going to affect the decision about the confirmatory test. Up till now, and according to what we heard in San Antonio during the AABB-meeting, most people are taking into account that the confirmatory test would be the Western blot method. Now in view of the crossreactivity, one may discuss again whether that is the most appropriate test, or whether perhaps we should look for reverse transcriptase as a confirmatory test. What is your opinion?

R.J. Gerety:

The crossreactivity is elicited in animals that are hyperimmunised. Presumably, crossreactivity of antibodies might be seen among populations that are repeatedly exposed to high-risk products, like hemophiliacs. The crossreactivity I describe is readily detectable on Western blot; it is against a single protein. With respect to your question concerning reverse transcriptase, I am very excited about it, but I am not sure how we can streamline the test as developed in our laboratory. Certainly, we were not trying to streamline it when we developed it; we wanted to be sure that we pelleted the virus and characterised it. It is a cumbersome, expensive test at present, but for screening for retrovirus I think it has the possibility of detecting them. It requires between 10^3 and 10^4 particles to be positive. So far, in collaboration with Dr. S. Iwarson, all 18 patients with non-A non-B hepatitis have had at least that number of particles, because they have all been positive in our test. It may function similarily to a hepatitis B antigen test, which is not very sensitive in terms of infectivity. There can be a thousand infectious hepatitis B viruses in a sample that is negative for surface antigen, but very few people have that low level of virus, most have considerably more. So, if it turns out that the retroviruses are present in reasonable numbers — as we have so far determined they are in 18 out of 18 non-A non-B hepatitis patients' sera — it will become a practical test from the standpoint of sensitivity. I think at this point the major problem is the mechanics of the test and its cost.

J. Goudsmit:

I think Dr. Gerety will agree that the reverse transcriptase is a confirmatory test for that specific antigen. So you have a problem, when you look for antibodies to HTLV-III and you do an RT assay as a confirmatory test. At that point you could only say that there is a retrovirus, but it could very well be another one than the one your antibody is directed against. So, then it is better to do the reverse transcriptase immediately instead of going through the anti HTLV-III antibody testing.

S. Iwarson:

Just to clarify the point of cross reactivity in the non-A non-B patients mentioned by Dr. Gerety. We looked for antibodies to HTLV-III by the ELISA technique in our non-A non-B patients but we did not find any.

J.B. Bussel:

Dr. Gerety, in regard to heat-treatment, is the non-A non-B virus equally, more or less susceptible to heat-treatment? Is there any data available on the preliminary studies that, I believe, Mannucci (3) among others are doing to investigate whether the heat-treatment inactivates non-A non-B?

R.J. Gerety:

We have done some studies to show that non-A non-B is inactivated by wet heat, which is the standard heat applied to stabilised albumins: 60°C for 10 hours. Data have also been presented that non-A non-B hepatitis can be inactivated by dry heat at varying temperatures for varying periods of time. With respect to non-A non-B hepatitis, I must say that the data are not ideal, because the amount of non-A non-B inactivated is unknown. Although the data are not wonderful, taken together they suggest that dry heat is effective for inactivating non-A non-B hepatitis. I think that the data Dr. Jason presented from the CDC suggested also that dry heat could inactivate HTLV-III. This stands in direct contrast to the clinical data that has been generated. There is evidence that there continues to be transmission of non-A non-B hepatitis, at least in terms of enzyme elevations that would appear to be associated with the infusion of the 'heat-treated' materials, some of which were subjected to wet heat and some dry heat. There is a dilemma at this point. You can hypothesise several things: That there is more than one agent, there is C and D and the chimpanzee is not susceptible to D. We could have a theoretical discussion, but the data suggest that dry heat inactivates HTLV-III as well as non-A non-B. We then have to explain the enzyme elevations in recipients of heat-treated material. It could be unrelated to infectivity, but from the data that I have seen, one would be hardpressed not to conclude that it was non-A non-B hepatitis. There is no biopsy confirmation, however. You are dealing strictly with enzyme elevations, but you are also dealing with newly diagnosed hemophiliacs who are young, who do no usually exhibit symptomatic hepatitis and yet the enzyme elevations are fairly consistent.

J.M. Jason (Atlanta):

Mannucci in Parma presented data on what is called virgin hemophiliacs, who had not received any therapy prior to the study (3). These people were started on heat-treated American factor concentrates and had been followed a year. Reportedly, they do not show signs of antibodies by Western blot to HTLV-III, which supports the idea that heat-treatment is effective against HTLV-III.

3. Rouzioux C, Chamaret S, Montagnier L, Carnelli V, Rolland G, Mannucci PM. Absence of antibodies to AIDS virus in haemophiliacs treated with heat-treated factor VIII concentrate. Lancet 1985;i:271-2.

J.B. Bussel:

Dr. Dichtelmüller, my understanding is that in the United States, it is very unlikely, though perhaps this is completely wrong that, the Office of Biologics would approve β-propiolactone ultraviolet treatment. Is that wrong and if it is not, what are the dangers of this treatment that would lead them to have had that opinion in the past, even if they do not have it in the present?

H. Dichtelmüller (Frankfurt am Main):

There is a point in treatment with β-propiolactone (βPL), the carcinogenic effect. But we have never detected any residual of βPL in the final product (4) βPL is degraded with a half life time of ~2.8 min in aqueous solutions, thus it depends simply on the time to eliminate βPL.

In my opinion there are no dangers in βPL treatment. Additionally, the virus inactivation is very effective, and we have two βPL-treated products under clinical study in the United States.

H.H. Gunson:

The prospects of screening donors for anti HTLV-III fills me with a certain amount of concern, because this is going to put an enormous cost onto the blood services. Should we not be concentrating on the final materials? I can see we are going to be screening all donors and yet the products are going to be heat-treated anyway. Why not just concentrate on getting the final material that is free and use the test for batches of that, rather than for every donor that contributes to the pool?

J.M. Jason:

I will initiate, although Dr. Gerety will be the more definitive commentor from the U.S.A. side. All of these assays, for instance, the one I showed, while being very sensitive theoretically, still do not exclude the presence of viral particles. Clearly, the results concerning heat-treatment are very comforting — that something can be done very quickly, even before donor screening becomes widely available. But for true insurance sake, it is always better to have a backup in regard to donor screening.

R.J. Gerety:

If you do not know about and cannot detect virus in plasma derivatives, then you can treat it in a manner to inactivate viruses, in general. But if you know a way to prevent a virus from entering a plasma pool, I think you have to do that even if it is expensive.

4. Pruggmayer D, Stephan W. Gas chromatographic trace analysis of β-propiolactone in sterilised serum proteins. Vox Sang 1976;31:191-8.

J.M. Jason:

But again a note of caution from the other side. At least for an antibody assay; it appears from the chimpanzee studies that it may take 3 or 4 months for sero-conversion. So a negative test does not guarantee that that person is non-infectious.

J. Goudsmit:

The other thing, which was mentioned is that you cannot use an anti-body test for screening the final pools, because there you are interested in antigen. As soon as you have an antigen test, you can screen as well the donor pool for antigen. But we are not at that stage, yet.

R.A. Coutinho:

The other side of the coin, of course, is what do you tell the donor. Does anyone have any ideas about this?

R.J. Gerety:

As I said, by the time we have finished with these large-scale clinical studies in the U.S.A., I think we are going to be able to tell sero-positive donors that they have been exposed and recovered, or have antibody and virus coexisting in the sera.

Not everyone who is asymptomatic and has antibody will have the virus. We are going to try to confirm this by cell cultures and by reverse transcriptase tests. To get back to the other question about why not just inactivate the final product: Some of us presented data today estimating the most hepatitis B virus that might be present in a plasma pool. That is because we know the effect of screening. When we talked about β-propiolactone and UV, data indicated that the most virus that could be present is 10 per ml if it is non-A non-B, and 1,000 per ml if it is hepatitis B. If you leave it as a total unknown, I am certain that contamination will overload the system, the heating will not be effective in removing all infectivity. It is the same with hepatitis B; when there was too much virus, no matter what inactivation methods or procedures you applied, it was not adequate.

H.H. Gunson:

That is not entirely consistent with what has happened. Albumin pre-parations have been extremely safe, since they have been pasteurised.

R.J. Gerety:

I think albumin is a different situation although it brings up a point that I wanted to make: We intentionally contaminated plasma pools with Rous sarcoma virus and tracked it during fractionation using reverse transcriptase to see where the virus distributes, just as we had done earlier with hepatitis B. It does not appear to end up in fraction II. I am not sure whether that is because the concentration of alcohol is reasonably high in fraction II, from which the IgG is prepared, or whether it is simply a characteristic of the compartmentalisation of these viruses. When compared to the reverse transcriptase activity in serum, about 30% was found in cryoprecipitate. No detectable reverse transcriptase was present in immune-globulin, so I am sure that is one of the products that we do not have to worry about in terms of inactivating viruses, but obviously we would like additional data.

H. Dichtelmüller:

Is it possible to have estimations about the infectious titres of HTLV-III present in plasma? As far as I know, there are not any titrations. Do you have an idea of the magnitude of titres, are they lower or higher than hepatitis B or non-A non-B?

R.J. Gerety:

I do not have that information; I am not sure anyone does. But the culture systems that we normally use are very insensitive. About 1,000 HTLV-III per lymphocyte is necessary to get a positive culture. So, a routine positive culture means that we are dealing with a virus count that is more than 1,000 per lymphocyte as you set up the test. Culture is relatively insensitive and reverse transcriptase is relatively insensitive; so, to get some idea about inactivation you have to deal with large numbers of infectious viruses to begin with. This is possible with HTLV-III, but not with non-A non-B hepatitis virus.

C.Th. Smit Sibinga:

We are slowly coming to the heart of the matter. What I can distile from Dr. Gerety's comments is the state of the art. First of all, we have to find out what the natural course of this disease is, what it means when somebody has a positive antibody test, and what impact that might have in the future. This will take at least five years, if we take into account the extent of the so-called incubation period of the disease to become overt. What might be the impact of antibody positivity or the absence of it (as there is a certain suspicion about this) on the eventual relation to blood transfusion or the transfusion of any blood product. That is the first thing we need to find out.

Still, the question remains: What are we going to do? Are we prepared to say anything or to do anything with those donors who come out with a positive test, without any symptomatology or any further anamnesis? That is a very crucial point. I think we are not yet prepared for that — at least not in this country. I sensed the same feeling at the AABB-meeting in San Antonio.

A question which I would like to raise in this respect is: There were described a number of cases related not to blood products in the sense of FVIII or FIX concentrates, but to other blood products, where donors have been traced from whom these patients had received blood products over the past five years. Some of these donors had symptoms of AIDS or AIDS-related complex or did belong to risk groups (5). What happened

5. Curran JW, Lawrence DN, Jaffe H et al. Acquired immuno deficiency syndrome (AIDS) associated with transfusions. New Eng J Med 1984; 310:69-75.

to the patients who received other blood components from the same donors, in the same period of time? Is there any information available about this? Second point: What happened to the hemophiliacs who received products out of the same batches, where one individual developed AIDS from? Has there been any tracing back of this? In a couple of European countries there has been an enormous consumption of United States products over the past 5-6 years, for instance Germany. Yet, there are only two hemophiliacs described so far in Germany, who have developed AIDS, one being a drugaddict as well.

J.M. Jason:

Concerning recipients of other blood products from a donor who has had one recipient later develop AIDS — there is an on-going collaborative study dealing with that issue. I do not think that they have any final results yet. It is an ongoing study across the U.S.A.: Trying to do exactly what you have in mind. You can imagine the cost of these studies, how time-consuming they are, and how concerned people have to be about the emotional effects on a patient being contacted, saying, "By the way, someone else who received a product from your same donor has come down with AIDS". It is not an easy study. Finding these people is hard enough, let alone dealing with that.

Your second question, I think I can give a fairly comforting response to, but it depends on whether you are an optimist or a pessimist. We spend a great deal of time tracking down lot numbers received by persons with hemophilia and AIDS. In this, you are dealing with the problem of denominators: How do you decide if something is significant or not. Happily, there were so many different lot numbers and so little overlap that it is highly unlikely that cases of AIDS were related to a given lot. There was only one lot that had been taken by 4 AIDS patients and the remainder of lots had been taken by at most 2 patients. That one particular lot taken by 4 patients clearly had a very wide distribution. So, trying to pinpoint specific lots becomes a little bit beyond the realm of reason. What we are now doing though is: There has been a number of lot withdrawls, because a donor later developed AIDS. The first three of those withdrawls were put into a collaborative study, where recipients were matched to people who were exposed to other lots. That study will be completed within the next couple of months. It was a massive study and we learned a great deal from it: Number one, that the hemophiliac community is very well organised and incredibly concerned about the problem. So, for no money, many health care providers and patients volunteered to help.

Number two, since one of the matching criteria was the factor dosage, we found that unfortunately, these volunteers did not know their patients' factor dosages very well. When we went to the records and got the actual dosages; they had nothing to do with what the caretakers thought the patients took. So we are now rematching. An unmatched analysis shows no difference between exposed and non-exposed persons in HTLV-III/LAV antibody prevalence, but again you are dealing with a high background rate of antibody positivity. There was no difference in immune function, except for PHA and Con A mitogen responses. However, until we do the matched analysis, I would take these data as preliminary. Within a few months we should have the results of this matched analysis.

R.J. Gerety:

We did rough calculations and feel that for every lot of FVIII that is produced in the United States an average of 100 people received this same product. So, if there is no lot association of the first 20 or so cases, then you can multiply that by 100 to indicate the number who were exposed.

R.L. McShine (Groningen):

Concerning the neutralisation of possible hepatitis B virus in blood products, I believe that for the production of these antibodies, some manufacturers use human plasma or serum as starting material. As we know, we do not have any test available for non-A non-B virus, and other retroviruses. Is there not a danger of transmitting non-A non-B virus or retroviruses in this material?

R.J. Gerety:

If I have understood you correctly, you are questioning whether or not the addition of specific antibody to neutralise virus might itself pose a threat for, for instance, non-A non-B hepatitis? I think that is a great deal less threat than the plasma-derived product itself, which is 100% contamined with non-A non-B hepatitis. I can tell you that now. As for immunoglobulins in general, we fractionated materials which contained a variety of retroviruses including some of the infectious sera that we use for non-A non-B hepatitis studies. There still is something magical about immunoglobulin, it does not contain infectious non-A non-B virus. We have not followed through, although we know it does not contain infectious Rous sarcoma virus when you contaminate the starting pool. I do not know at this point whether it is partitioning of virus or the alcohol concentration in fraction II, but it is not a high-risk product for transmission of disease, which confirms what we have known for some time about this product.

H.H. Gunson:

Can I just pick up this point, Dr. Gerety? Is that intramuscular immunoglobulin that you are talking about? Because a batch of intravenous immunoglobulin produced in England gave non-A non-B hepatitis to recipients.

R.J. Gerety:

That particular lot of immunoglobulin was treated quite differently. It began as fraction II powder, but it was put through column chromatography. One can add immunoglobulin to products which has not been altered to accomodate intravenous administration, however. Something analogous to this occurs each time you administer AHF which can easily contain 1 to 2% immunoglobulin as manufactured.

H.H. Gunson:

But it does indicate that the virus may be in the basic fraction II.

R.J. Gerety:

That is one interpretation. The other is that the column chromatography material, which had been used for other materials, was the source of the contamination and not the fraction II. That would be my interpretation of the data, although I think your point is well taken. Intravenous immunoglobulins which begin with fraction II may contain complexed antibody plus virus. You may dissociate it while you treat it to make it appropriate for intravenous use, and we are very concerned about that at present in the U.S.A.

F. Peetoom:

Dr. Jason, you added to your list the incidence of HTLV-III antibody in thalassemia and the sickle cell. These were not AIDS-cases, but antibody positives. Was this done to contrast the low incidence, in comparison with hemophilia? And if so, would you elaborate on the reasons that might be behind this, other than that they used all frozen washed red cells? Are you certain of that?

J.M. Jason:

They were chosen specifically as a comparison group, receiving frozen blood cells as opposed to concentrates. The purpose was initially not to contrast their sero-prevalence to HTLV-III; the initial study had been to look at their immune function. At that point, we felt that in addition to the problem of AIDS, the factor itself was immunosuppressive, and that the frozen red cells, in addition to just being cellular blood products and thus a potential route of infection, were also providing an antigenic load and were thus an important comparison group. The issue of direct immunosuppression by antigen load was thus another area we wanted to deal with, but things have moved faster than we expected and we were able to show the persons who received only FPRC did not have a high rate of antibody to HTLV-III.

J. Goudsmit:

Was there any geographic determinant in those patients? Because the background of that type of patients has presumably higher prevalence of HTLV-III seropositivity than other groups. Is this true?

J.M. Jason:

Yes. I mentioned it probably too quickly. They were all from the New York City area and received their cellular blood products from, in general, donors from that area.

J. Goudsmit:

What was their genetic or racial background?

J.M. Jason:

The sickle cell anemics were all black. In the thalassemias we have broken down to Mediterraneans and others, but basically white. They were all born in the U.S. and had not left the U.S.A. in the last five years, although many are of Mediterranean extraction.

F. Peetoom:

Dr. Jason, what is the current discussion on predisposition? There has been a lot of work done in the homosexual high-risk group in particular to identify if there were any predisposing practices, if you will. Since there are many people exposed to supposedly contaminated products, and some do and some do not develop AIDS, is it mainly a matter of dosage? Or, as you have demonstrated in your figures, that the more product the higher is the incidence? Or are there still other factors that are still assumed to be of predisposing nature, like immuno-suppression coinciding with exposure?

J.M. Jason:

I think you probably hit one of the most important questions for up-coming research. Especially in a population like people with hemophilia, you are now talking in the U.S.A. of 74% seropositivity. There are a couple of ways to look at that. One is a possible but pessimistic view-point that all those people could come down with full blown AIDS. We do know the incubation period is long. It appears to be a virus that will incorporate into the genome, so in addition to worrying about long incubation periods you really can also say that you are dealing with a latent virus. The only other thing to address now would be the issue of cofactors. If they are all not going to come down with AIDS, what will predict who will and how can you prevent it? That is certainly going to be a very important area to look at in the coming years.

S. Iwarson:

As you know there is a discussion going on that you must have a stimulated lymphocyte to have a target cell for HTLV-III.

P.B.A. Kernoff (London):

We have heard that around 80% of heavily treated hemophiliacs — at least those treated with U.S.A. commercial products — are positive for anti HTLV-III. We also know that a large proportion of these patients have chronic abnormalities of liver function tests. I have heard it argued that there is not much point in using heat-treated or sterilised products to treat these patients, because they have already been exposed. I wonder whether the panel has any views on that?.

J.M. Jason:

It gets back to the issue relating to what antibody status means. You do not know whether a portion of those people have been immunised, whether they are infected, or what is going on. If you know that certain material is contaminated and that something can be done to decrease or prevent the contamination, there is every reason to do something about it; not just for those who are still antibody negative, but if repeated exposure as a cofactor is present, be it via activation or some other mechanism, the cleaner the better.

R.J. Gerety:

I think that was well spoken, It is the same question that was asked in another form before. If you have noted that someone is infected, why not give him the same virus again? I do not know what that means. That may be a lot worse for that patient. I think once you know that there is a virus contamination and you know how to remove it, then you have to remove it.

W.G. van Aken:

Dr. Coutinho, I believe it is fair to say that I have not received an answer to my question which I asked earlier. I do not blame the panel for that, because I think it is a very difficult question to answer: What shall we tell the positive donor? I know that you are personally involved in a study in Amsterdam among male homosexuals in which you are doing a follow-up study on the prevalence of anti-HTLV/LAV.

What are you telling those homosexuals when they have a positive test? We can learn from that how to develop a policy with relation to the donors.

R.A. Coutinho:

In this study all are voluntary participants and the idea is to tell them the results of the test, unless someone says in advance that he does not want to know it. We will tell them that we do not know exactly what it means. We presume that the people who participate in this trial would want to know exactly their immunological parameters and also their serological status. We will inform both the participant and the general pratitioner.

J.M. Jason:

It might help if I mention what is going on with the hemophiliac patients. The point that has just been made is the most important one: These are people participating in a study. Unfortunately, that is not the boat you are going to be in with donors. We have now sent out triple-checked results to all the physicians with patients collaborating in these studies, with a letter that had been in part worked out with CDC lawyers concerning what should be told to the patients. The gist of it is to do whatever you do in person: To sit down with them and explain that nothing is known about the meaning of a positive test or a negative test, and remind them that that is the reason, in fact, the study is being done.

With hemophiliacs again, it is much easier because you have a group of people who half expected what the result would be. It is not quite the burden it is going to be on donors. What you do find is concern about their household and what risk there is to their household members.

184

C.Th. Smit Sibinga:

Mr. Chairman, could I pick up the thread again and come back to Prof. van Aken's question, which bothers me as well, of course, as a blood banker being responsible for a certain area in this country. It relates in a sense to one of the other provocative statements of Dr. Goudsmit. He stated that hemophiliacs preferably should be treated with cryo-precipitates. I do not agree. Apparently, he is not a hemophiliac himself and he does not have a son with hemophilia. We should try to treat our patients with local products. Not that we know what the incidence of the virus of the antibody is in our population, we have not even started testing. But this does not necessarily mean that it will prevent them from getting AIDS. I think if we want to get started in trying to prevent blood borne AIDS as effective as possible, according to the state of the art, there are basically four fronts which we should open:

One is already open: To try to convince our donor population as well as possible that they have a moral obligation towards the recipient (6) in making clear to us whether they think they belong to any risk category or not, and not to come to the centre just to obtain the knowledge as to whether or not they are carriers of something.

The second front is: Could we do any test on those who were not self-excluded from the program, so those who donate the blood? What actually should we do then? For the time being, I understand that an antibody test might give at least some information to unravel some of the mysteries surrounding this disease. There is a certain future for an antigen test, a virus test. Here we have a problem: Which of the antigens are we going to test; and what does it mean? Is it an envelope, is it a core? What are the infective parts presented in the test?

The third front is: The reduction of the pool size. That is the essence of the treatment with cryoprecipitate. Could we reduce the risk by reducing the pool size, the number of donors contributing to the eventual final pool for our product? That is an important thing, but there is more related to the product than just the pool size. There is the quality, there is the specific activity, the concentration, the ease of handling, the comfort for the patient's life. These are very important aspects which you should take into account.

Finally: There are efforts — we have heard evidence today of the success of these efforts — to eventually inactivate this threatening virus through heattreatment, either in the wet state or in the dry state. We know that the dry state might be even more effective and might less intensively jeopardise the already poor yields of the final product: FVIII.

F. Peetoom:

Depending on how many specifically positive HTLV-III antibody donors are going to be found, we are for some years going to create a growing inventory of concerned, anxious and frightened people. Not just frightened for themselves, but frightened about their role within their families, with their children or spouses, their employment, how they will be considered in other social environments. These people indeed are at risk of identifying themselves with pariahs. Some will more than others,

6. Hantchef ZS. The development of blood transfusion and its ethical, legislative and economic impact. Transfusion Newsletter 1977;11/12: 3-4.

but I have already seen many people with a tremendous range of anxiety levels that require a lot of our attention. The medical director of a Blood Bank is obviously not available enough hours in the day to deal effectively with this growing inventory of people, who want to know not just information this time, but what is evolving, what could give them more reassurance. We are considering having a specially trained registered nurse for psychological counselling and support to deal with these donors, and, if necessary, select additional professional support.

R.A. Coutinho:

The point is where the responsibility of the Blood Bank ends.

J. Goudsmit:

I think one of the important point is: If the testing for HTLV-III antibodies will be mainly done by Blood Banks, you are in trouble. As soon as other laboratories in the country will do it as well, then you have another situation. I see that problem very well. If only the Blood Banks are doing this test, you will solicit certain persons who will come mainly to know their antibody status. When certain assays are available for testing, they will be used by other laboratories as well. At that point, a lot of those questions will be channelled through these routes.

W.G. van Aken:

Dr. Jason, did I get you right, that there may be a difference between the prevalence of AIDS in hemophilia A and hemophilia B? And that that may be related to a cofactor? You had indicated that there were differences in the subpopulations of the lymphocytes between hemophilia A and hemophilia B patients. Could you very briefly speculate on what sort of mechanism may be behind those differences?

J.M. Jason:

For the incidence of AIDS, there is really no statistical difference, given the lower incidence of hemophilia B in the general population. However, there is a very significant difference in antibody prevalence. One of the possible explanations for the data I showed on T helper-cell numbers is that in fact some of the FIX patients may not be infected. Some may be immunised, so what you see with the higher T helper-cell numbers are people that are immunised and not infected. It takes us into an area of work that we are right now active in. Data which I did not show, indicate that between FVIII recipients, FIX recipients and AIDS-patients there is a very different pattern of antibodies in regard to what antigens these people have antibodies to. Initially, I was very excited because I thought it might represent a difference between being infected and being immunised. We found a much lower prevalence of antibody to the surface antigen P-41 in the FIX recipients. But if you look at the association between the different antibodies and T helper-cell numbers, it does not fit with that hypothesis. So now, my second hypothesis is: We are really picking up different points in sero-conversion. It is a bit like hepatitis B or EBV — you pick up different antibodies at different points in time and that is being reflected in these trends. We are now testing serial samples on homosexual lymphadenopathy patients to see if we can pull that apart.

IV. Clinical aspects

NEEDS, QUALITY VERSUS QUANTITY

S. Seidl

INTRODUCTION

Human plasma is used as the starting material for the preparation of several blood products which are used under various clinical circumstances: Albumin, coagulation factor preparations and immunoglobulins. A sophisticated organization is required to provide plasma products in sufficient amounts. This is accomplished by national or regional blood transfusion services or by commercial companies. In many countries, such as the Federal Republic of Germany both systems do exist. However, most of the factor VIII concentrates and immunoglobulin preparations are provided by pharmaceutical companies.

In this paper some clinical aspects of these plasma derivatives with reference to the source material needed will be summarized, whereas a detailed discussion of these preparations will be given by the following authors.

The headline of this presentation is "quality versus quantity". These two terms however, are not always antagonistic. From the clinical point of view both quantity as well as quality have to be taken into account. This is best illustrated by factor VIII preparations. Wastage of source material has been defined by the ISBT Working Party on "Socio-Economic Aspects of Blood Transfusion", if plasma is processed into factor VIII preparations with a yield of less than 200 IU/kg of starting material. (1) In terms of hepatitis safety, however, improvement of quality is required. This has resulted in factor VIII preparations containing less than 10% of the original factor VIII content. Both preparations are in clinical use and both are needed.

REQUIREMENTS FOR SOURCE MATERIAL

For the preparation of plasma derivatives a technology is required that guarantees a reproducible and standardized preparation. In order to achieve this a defined source material is needed. Although this has already been discussed in the beginning of this symposium I would like to re-emphasize these problems, referring in particular to my own country. Requirements for raw material have been published by national and international health authorities or by scientific societies. Several years ago the German Society for Blood Transfusion and Immunohaematology has established a task force which dealt with these problems and formulated minimum requirements for source plasma (2). Tests which have to be performed on single donor plasma or pool plasma include serum protein content, screening for HBsAg (on single donor plasma) by radioimmunoassay (RIA) or enzymeimmunoassay (ELISA), bacteriological control of the source material, protein analysis by electrophoresis and immunoelectrophoresis, hemoglobin concentration in the source plasma, no pyrogenicity, a check for identity (positive reaction against human serum by immuneprecipitation) and compatibility (using animal experiments). If the source material is lyophilized the moisture content must also be determined.

From January 1st, 1985, the Federal Health Office of the German Federal Republic may require additional anti-HBc testing for human plasma used for factor VIII production. By this procedure the potential risk of transmitting AIDS through blood transfusion should be minimized, although anti-HBc testing is in no way a specific test to detect carriers of HTLV-III. Even though the discovery of the probable cause of AIDS has resulted in much less interest in non-specific tests in general this "surrogate test" may be considered as an appropriate means of identifying members of high risk groups, thus additionally reducing the risk of transmitting AIDS by blood or blood products. As a result of this anti-HBc screening the amount of source plasma will be reduced and likely approximately 20-30.000 litres of fresh plasma will not be used for factor VIII preparations. This corresponds to an overall frequency of 8% anti-HBc positive donors. Removal of anti-HBc positive donors may lead to product shortages and price increases. If anti-HBc positive plasma could be used for other purposes (albumin, production of reagents) the cost impact would be less unfavourable. Nevertheless, the implementation of anti-HBc testing would increase the costs for testing (staff, discard of positive units if not used for other preparations and recruitment efforts to replace anti-HBc positive donors).

On the other hand the fractionation industry has voluntarily withdrawn coagulation products manufactured from pools containing plasma from donors who developed AIDS subsequent to donation. It also became evident that in all these instances donors were identified as members of a high risk groups, i.e. the withdrawal would not have taken place if members of high risk groups had not been excluded. It should also be kept in mind that each withdrawal has severe economical consequences and has even more severe physical consequences for hemophiliacs who utilized this product prior to withdrawal. Each such withdrawal therefore, also has an effect on the supply of coagulation factors.

A specific test for AIDS is anticipated in the near future, which then may replace anti-HBc testing. It has been shown by a enzyme-linked immunosorbent assay (ELISA) that most patients with AIDS have antibodies against the retrovirus which causes AIDS (LAV or HTLV-III). It is also interesting to note that a higher frequency of LAV antibodies was discovered in hemophiliacs treated with high doses of factor VIII concentrates than in those patients receiving lower amounts of factor VIII.

FACTOR VIII PREPARATIONS

Since the introduction of the cryoprecipitation technique for harvesting factor VIII, much work has been done to improve the purity of factor VIII without affecting its clotting activity. Several products are now available.

Cryoprecipitates. This can be prepared as frozen cryoprecipitate in almost all blood centers, but has the principal disadvantage that it is not feasible to assay factor VIII concentration of each unit. Therefore, an assumed value has to be taken which must be set with care because the great individual variation in potency may result in wastage of the product due to excess therapy or in low in vivo levels and continued bleeding due to inadequate therapy. A yield of 400 IU/kg plasma may be obtained which is in terms of quantity, an excellent result.

Small pool freeze-dried cryoprecipitates are preparations consisting of 8 to 12 plasma donations. This product has still a high yield of factor VIII (300 IU/kg starting plasma) and has the further advantage that storage, transportation and stability are considerably better. In developing countries this product can be used for home-therapy thus providing adequate care for a large number of hemophiliacs spread over a wide geographical area.

Factor VIII concentrates are prepared from multiple donations of fresh plasma. The final product contains freeze-dried material of known potency. This product has the advantage that a defined amount of coagulation factor VIII is transfused. It is therefore possible to predict the number of international units of factor VIII required to achieve hemostasis in a particular clinical situation. Furthermore, the volume to be injected is smaller which makes these preparations suitable for home-therapy. Two preparations are in use: Intermediate purity concentrates and concentrates of high purity.

The price to be part for purification and concentration of factor VIII is its high loss of coagulation activity in the fractionation process. The practical question which arises is how far can transfusion services and donor community go to meet the demand. However, the situation with respect to hemophilia is only one of several examples of the growing clinical demand for more and better blood products. As each major speciality introduces intensive and sophisticated methods of clinical management, each blood bank will be confronted with new and increasing demands for highly purified blood components.

Intermediate purity concentrates: Factor VIII concentrates of intermediate purity are prepared from large pools of plasma. Yields of 200 IU/kg source plasma can be obtained when careful attention is paid to blood collection and plasma separation procedures.

High purity concentrates too can be obtained only at the expense of yield, resulting in approximately 100 IU/kg of starting material. This product has several advantages, i.e. improved solubility, reduction in fibrinogen content and low concentrations of iso-agglutinins.

The main risk attached to the use of factor VIII concentrates of human origin is the transmission of viral hepatitis. It is a well-known fact, that many hemophiliacs suffer from hepatitis infection. In recent years factor VIII concentrates have been made available which are considered to be free from transmitting hepatitis and other transmissible diseases. A factor VIII preparation, highly purified and heated in solution, free of coagulable protein and immunoglobulin is in clinical use. The efficacy of pasteurization was tested in chimpanzees with a solution deliberately contaminated with infectious hepatitis B virus. Transfusion of pasteurized factor VIII concentrates did not transmit hepatitis to chimpanzees. The clinical follow up of these concentrates over 5 years showed no case of hepatitis B infection in patients. However, this special treatment results in a further decrease of the factor VIII related to source plasma is only about 8% (3).

Although it might be desirable to treat all hemophiliacs with hepatitis safe preparations, the amount of source material needed should also be taken into consideration. The ISBT Working Party or "Socio-Economic Aspects of Blood Transfusion" has pointed out the importance of equitable treatment in the management of hemophilia, which requires careful resource management. If has been generally accepted that the principles of cost-effectiveness apply in the processing of factor VIII preparations.

Although general agreement has been reached on the amounts required, with a minimum of 20,000 IU of factor VIII per annum for all diagnosed severe hemophiliacs, adequate treatment of many hemophiliacs may involve significantly larger volumes of factor VIII (4). In some countries the average of factor VIII per hemophiliac exceeds 50,000 IU/ year.

The availability of source plasma can be increased considerably if the clinical use of the fresh frozen plasma decreases. At the present time the German Red Cross Blood Transfusion Centers collect more than 2 Million donations per year, approximately two-third of the blood is transfused as red cell concentrates. However, it has been estimated that not more than one-third of the present needs for factor VIII can be provided from local sources because (i) large amounts of source plasma are still used as fresh frozen plasma and (ii) the separated plasma has to be frozen within 6 hours.

The effect of delayed processing on factor VIII activity has been well documented. When plasma is stored, factor VIII activity initially decreases fast but becomes more stable after some time. Experiences from West-Germany have shown that also from this "old" plasma (stored for approximately 18 hours after collection) up to 300 IU/kg source plasma can be harvested. The utilization of this plasma for factor VIII preparation would considerably increase the amount of source material.

Other variables which influence the quality of fresh frozen plasma are the composition of the anticoagulant and the speed of freezing, whereas the storage temperature (-20° or -40°C) did not significantly alter the factor VIII content (5). The poor recovery of factor VIII in ACD or CPD is due, in part, to the marked instability of the factor VIII molecule. It has been shown that the presence of calcium affects the molecular organization which influences the cryoprecipitability. Since heparin inhibits clot formation by preventing the action of thrombin the ionic consumption is changed, in particular physiological levels of calcium are maintained. In several sets of experiments it could be demonstrated, that the recovery of factor VIII was significantly greater in heparin plasma than in CPD plasma (6,7). Heparin is not suitable for red cell storage. However, Smit Sibinga and co-workers have shown that the addition of CPD anticoagulant to these red cells results in a normal storage time (8).

Factor VIII is also available from non-human sources. Pig blood is particularly rich in factor VIII and a clinically acceptable high purity procine factor VIII is used for treatment of patients with an inhibitor. Although the animal protein is immunogenic to man, many patients have not developed antibodies or shown only low titred antibody.

The present discussion on adequate factor VIII supply may be radically affected by further progress in recombinant DNA technology which may provide factor VIII from an alternative source. The first successful steps have already been reported. A factor VIII cDNA was transferred into a mammalian cell line which now synthesises and secretes human factor VIII. Such a breakthrough, if commercially available, will have tremendous impact on the fractionation industry.

FACTOR IX CONCENTRATES

This coagulation factor is less labile than factor VIII and approximately 80% of the original factor IX activity may still be present in whole blood after 3 weeks of storage. Nevertheless fresh plasma is a more reliable source of factor IX for the preparation of concentrates. These concentrates are prepared by ion-exchange chromatography on cellulose or

Sephadex A 50. Factor IX concentrates are used for the treatment of patients with hemophilia B (Christmas disease). A therapeutic dose is injected intravenously by a syringe which is advantageous when compared with fresh frozen plasma. The latter necessitates administration by continuous intravenous infusion due to the low level of factor IX in this preparation.

Factor IX concentrates sometimes do not contain sufficient amounts of factor VII and those concentrates are not effective in the treatment of hemorraghic complications in severe liver disease. Therefore, factor VII has to be administered which usually requires large volumes of fresh frozen plasma.

Hepatitis safe preparation of factor IX (PPSB) are also available. They are prepared from β-propiolactone/UV-treated human plasma resulting in approximately 50% loss of factor IX activity. By this "cold-sterilization" procedure hepatitis B virus titers are reduced about 10^7-fold, whereas the reduction of infectivity by pasteurization is 10^4-fold (4). Recent experiments demonstrated that the combined treatment (β-PL/UV) is also effective in inactivating hepatitis non-A non-B viruses and some retroviruses. Neither case reports nor prospective clinical trials and chimpanzee studies revealed transmission of hepatitis.

FIBRONECTIN

This plasma protein has been identified as an opsonic mediator of the clearance function of the reticuloendothelial system (RES). Its main biological properties are the influence of phagocytosis because fibronectin promotes the binding of phagocytic material to macrophages. It also has interaction with fibrin and factor VIII.

Evaluation of fibronectin levels in several diseases have shown that a deficit may be associated with disseminated intravascular coagulation, severe trauma, and sepsis. So far the reported benefits of fibronectin suppletion by cryoprecipitate infusion are controversial (9) although the firbonectin level has been increased (10). At the present time the clinical effects of fibronectin treatment are still doubtfull and further controlled trials are urgently needed.

Fibronectin may be prepared by the precipitation method, using cryoprecipitate as the source material. This procedure includes reprecipitation of the dissolved cryoprecipitate, and addition of albumin. Fibronectin is stored after lyophilization. As the cryoprecipitates are made of outdated plasma, fibronection production does not interfere with factor VIII production. Also affinity chromatography may be used for fibronectin production. Elution from gelatin Sepharose 4 B with 8 M urea seems to be the appropriate buffer to obtain a non-denaturated product.

IMMUNOGLOBULIN PREPARATIONS

Immunoglobulins are valuable and increasingly used therapeutic products. Their clinical efficacy has been demonstrated in patients suffering from antibody deficiency and recently also in patients suffering from auto-immune disaeses, i.e. the effective treatment of ITP and possibly some other autoantibody mediated diseases. Most preparations produced by the Cohn method are only recommended for intramuscular administration, because adverse reactions following intravenous injections are linked to anticomplement activity, due to the presence of aggregated IgG.

For i.v. immunoglobulins several modifications have been introduced. Enzymatic treatment with pepsin or plasmin which results in IgG fragments, accompanied with intact 7 S IgG. Chemically modified IgG (treatment with β-propiolactone, reduced and alkylated, or sulfonated), immunoglobulins isolated with PEG, and "non-modified" preparations which are treated at pH 4.0. Remarkable differences have been observed concerning the half-life of IgG after injection, but all preparations demonstrate a good compatibility as shown by a low non-specific complement activation.

For the preparation of specific i.v. immunoglobulins also collumn ion exchange chromatography has been used. With a DEAE-Sephadex chromatographic process many thousands of vials of anti-D immunoglobulins have been prepared and intravenously injected. This procedure allows the recovery of substantial amounts of antibodies from hyperimmune plasma. Analysis of IgG and antibody recoveries demonstrated antibody activities between 50 and 90%. The immunoglobulin appeared to have a somewhat altered heavy-chain IgG subclass distribution which may account for the varying efficacy of recovery of different antibodies (11). The antibodies contain IgG_1 and IgG_3 in rather large amounts and these subclasses are recovered in highest yield (91%). The recovery of rabies antibodies and varicella zoster antibodies was much less (71% and 56%, respectively). These percentages are very close to the total IgG content (69% and 62%) thus demonstrating that the antibodies may be distributed equally between each subclass (11). Recently the effect of anti CMV IgG treatment of patients after bone marrow transplantation has been tested in a randomized study performed in several bone marrow transplantation centres. It could be demonstrated that the i.v. administration of anti-CMV IgG modifies both CMV disease and mortality (12). Apart from these severely immunosuppressed patients CMV also causes significant morbidity and mortality in small sick premature infants and splenectomized multitransfused patients or patients receiving granulocyte transfusions.

Blood transfusion services can contribute to the prevention of transfusion transmitted CMV infection by providing CMV negative blood and blood components (granulocytes) and, which might be even more important, by collecting plasma with high-titre CMV antibody for the CMV immunoglobulins (13).

REFERENCES

1. Beal RW. Socio-Economic Aspects of Blood Transfusion. Vox Sang 1984;46(suppl.1):104-7.
2. German Society of Blood Transfusion and Immunohaematology. Task Force for Requirements of Source Plasma, Frankfurt am Main, 1977.
3. Heimburger N, Schwinn H, Gratz P, Kumpe G, Herchenhans B. A factor VIII concentrate, highly purified and heated in solution. Abstract Ist International Haemophilia Conference, Bonn, 1980.
4. Stephan W, Dichtelmüller H, Kotitschke R, Prince AM, Friis RR, Bauer H. Inactivation of hepatitis viruses (B, non-A/non-B) and retroviruses in pooled human plasma by means of β-propiolactone and uv-treatment. Abstracts 18th Congress of the International Society of Blood Transfusion, Karger, Basel 1984:76.
5. Koerner K, Stampe D. Die Stabilität von Faktoren des Gerinnungssystems im tiefgefrorenen Frischplasma während der Lagerung bei -20°C und -40°C. Infusionstherapie 1984;11:46-50.

6. Rock GA, Cruickshank WH, Tackberry ES, Palmer DS. Improved yields of factor VIII from heparinized plasma. Vox Sang 1979;36: 290-300.
7. Smit Sibinga CTh, Welbergen H, Das PC. High-yield method of production of freeze-dried purified factor VIII by Blood Banks. The Lancet, 1981;ii:449-50.
8. De Jonge J, Smit Sibinga CTh, Das PC. Metabolic aspects and viability of heparin/CPDA-1 stored red cell concentrates as a by-product of a high yield factor VIII production method. Haemostasis 1983;13:214-8.
9. Lundsgaard-Hansen P. Plasma fibronectin in anaesthesiology and intensive care. Abstract 18th Congress of the International Society of Blood Transfusion, Karger, Basel 1984:45.
10. Hesselvik F, Brodin B, Carlsson C, Jorfeldt L, Lieden G, Cedergren B. Cryoprecipitate therapy in hyperdynamic septic shock – a controlled clinical study. Abstract 18th Congress of the International Society of Blood Transfusion. Karger, Basel 1984:46.
11. Friesen AD, Bowman IM, Bels WCH. Column ion exchange chromatographic production of human immune globulins and albumin. In: Separations of plasma proteins. Curling JM ed., Pharmacia Fine Chemicals AB, Uppsala, Sweden 1983:118-25.
12. Wernet P. Cytomegalovirus infection after allogeneic bone marrow transplantation. Abstracts 18th Congress of the International Society of Blood Transfusion. Karger, Basel 1984:57.
13. Contreras M. CMV and blood transfusion. Abstracts 18th Congress of the International Society of Blood Transfusion, Karger Basel 1984:57.

CLINICAL CHARACTERISTICS OF THE FACTOR VIII PROTEIN FROM VARIOUS FACTOR VIII CONCENTRATES

I.M. Nilsson

INTRODUCTION

Since factor VIII concentrates are necessary for the treatment not only of patients with hemophilia A but also for those with von Willebrand's disease, it is important to know all factor VIII related activities contained in the various concentrates now available.

We have studied factor VIII related activities in a number of factor VIII concentrates including cryoprecipitates, fraction I-O, intermediate and high purity preparations, heat treated concentrates and also concentrates prepared from plasma obtained from DDAVP stimulated blood donors. The in vivo properties of seven concentrates were studied in 10 hemophiliacs after infusion of comparable doses.

MATERIALS AND METHODS

Factor VIII concentrates (Table 1)

AHF-Kabi (human fraction I-O) prepared according to the Blombäck and Blombäck glycine method (1,2).

DDAVP AHF-Kabi. Plasma from donors stimulated by DDAVP intranasally (0.25 ml of DDAVP, Ferring, containing 1300 µg/ml) one hour before blood collection, was used (3). Otherwise, the preparation procedure was the same as for AHF-Kabi.

Octonativ (Kabi). Cryoprecipitate is used as starting material. The further purification procedure includes $Al(OH)_3$ adsorption, and the removal of fibrinogen by heparin-Sepharose.

DDAVP Octonativ (Kabi). Plasma from donors stimulated by DDAVP intranasally (see DDAVP AHF-Kabi).

Hemofil (Hyland). Cryoprecipitate is used as starting material. Fibrinogen is removed by polyethylene glycol, and factor VIII precipitated by adding glycine.

Hemofil T (Hyland). Prepared in the same way as Hemofil except that heat treatment of the freeze-dried product has been included.

Factorate Generation II or Factorate High Purity (Armour). Cryoprecipitate is used as starting material. Further purification includes $Al(OH)_3$ adsorption, cold ethanol precipitation, and re-suspension in citrate-glycine solution.

Kryobulin (Immuno). Cryoprecipitate is used as starting material; the preparation is then further purified by partial removal of fibrinogen.

Profilate (Alpha). Cryoprecipitate is used as starting material. Further purification includes $Al(OH)_3$ adsorption, and the removal of fibrinogen by polyethylene glycol (4.5%). Factor VIII is first precipitated by polyethylene glycol (15%), then dissolved and precipitated once again by glycine.

Profilate HS (Alpha). Profilate heat treated in solution.

Criostat (Laboratorios Grifols S.A.). Cryoprecipitate is used as starting material. The further purification procedure includes $Al(OH)_3$ adsorption,

Table 1. The factor VIII concentrates studied, data given by manufacturers.

	No. of batches	Preparation procedure	1 bottle 1 ampoule volume	Units VIII:C	Protein mg/ml
AHF-Kabi	5	Fraction I-0	100	270-290	18-24
DDAVP AHF-Kabi	1	Prepared from donors given DDAVP i.n.	100	445	15
Octonativ, Kabi	5	Cryoprec + $Al(OH)_3$ ads + removal of fib by hep-seph	10	455-525	21-30
DDAVP Octonativ, Kabi	2	Prepared from donors given DDAVP i.n.	10	776-1120	28-40
Hemofil, Hyland	5	Cryoprec + PEG + glycine prec	30	950-1200	20-30
Hemofil T, Hyland	5	Heat treated Hemofil	10	300	20
Factorate, Armour Generation II	2	Cryoprec + $Al(OH)_3$ ads + ethanol frac + extract with citrate glycine	50	1655-2025	9-13
Kryobulin, Immuno	2	Cryoprec + furhter purification	10	500	10-20
Profilate, Alpha	4	Cryoprec + $Al(OH)_3$ ads + PEG + glycine prec	25	690-880	20-25
Profilate HS, Alpha	1	Heat treated Profilate	25	500	40
AHF, Laboratories Grifols S.A.: Criostat	2	Cryoprec + $Al(OH)_3$ ads + PEG + ext with citrate-glycine	20	500	14-16
Criostat IP	2	Cryoprec + $Al(OH)_3$ ads	20	500	39-41
Criopecipitado	2	Cryoprec	10	150	75
Kryo-AHG, Finish Red Cross	2	Cryoprec	25	200	40
AHF-20; Intermediate Finnish Red Cross	1	Cryoprec + $Al(OH)_3$ ads	10	200	27

and the removal of fibrinogen by polyethylene glycol precipitation (4.5%). Factor VIII is precipitated by a higher concentration of polyethylene glycol (13%), and dissolved in glycine citrated saline to which dextrose and glycine have been added.

Criostat IP (laboratorios Grifols S.A.). Cryoprecipitate adsorbed with $Al(OH)_3$.

Crioprecipitado (Laboratorios Grifols S.A.). Freeze-dried cryoprecipitate.

Kryo-AHG (Finnish Red Cross). Freeze-dried cryoprecipitate.

AHF-20 Intermediate (Finnish Red Cross). Cryoprecipitate adsorbed by $Al(OH)_3$.

ASSAYS

Factor VIII clotting activity (VIII:C) assays.

1. One-stage assay. VIII:C activity was assessed from the normalizing effect on the recalcification time of platelet-rich hemophilia A plasma containing less than 1% VIII:C of the normal VIII:C concentration (4,5). Clotting time was read in a Photocoagulater (Kabi). Concentrates were diluted with saline until their activities corresponded to those of standard plasma, and then tested in 3 dilutions. The assays were carried out according to the balanced design described by Nilsson et al. (6).
2. Chromogenic VIII:C assay (Coatest, Kabi). This was performed as described by Rosén (7), bovine factors IXa and X and the chromogenic substrate S-2222 being used. The concentrates were prediluted with 0.05 M Tris buffer (pH 7.3) until their activities corresponded to those of standard plasma, and were then tested in a dilution of 1/80.

Two standards were used:
1. Pooled citrated plasma from 20 normal individuals, which was calibrated against the 9th British Standard plasma for factor VIII (79/504).
2. Concentrate standard (Kabi house standard No. Lss 10) previously calibrated against the 3rd International Standard for Blood Coagulation Factor VIII Human (80/556). Results were expressed as IU/ml. The pooled plasma was used as reference throughout the study for all types of assays.

Factor VIII coagulant antigen (VIII:CAg). This was assayed using a two-site solid phase immunoradiometric method (IRMA), based on one hemophilic antibody against VIII:C (8).

Factor VIII related antigen (VIIIR:Ag) was assayed using Laurell's immunielectrophoretic method (EIA), as described by Holmberg and Nilsson (9), and by immunoradiometric assay (IRMA) (10,11).

Factor VIII ristocetin cofactor activity (VIIIR:RCF) was assessed by a method using formalin fixed platelets (12), and results were expressed in U/ml.

The multimeric distribution of VIIIR:Ag was analyzed in concentrates by thin layer agarose electrophoresis in the presence of SDS, using a discontinuous buffer system according to a method described by Ruggeri and Zimmmerman (13). The bands corresponding to the multimers were identified in gels by reaction with ^{125}I-labeled affinity purified antibodies (rabbit anti-human VIIIR:Ag), followed by autoradiography. The concentrates were prediluted in 0.01 M Tris, 0.001 M EDTA, 2% SDS, pH 8.0 to about 1 U/ml and then tested in dilution 1:20.

Fibrinogen. This was assayed with a syneresis method (14).

Protein in the preparations was determined according to Blombäck and Blombäck (1).

Clinical material

The in vivo and biological half-life of various concentrates (AHF-Kabi, Octonativ, DDAVP Octonativ, Hemofil, Hemofil T, Profilate, Profilate HS) were evaluated after intravenous injection into 10 patients with severe hemophilia A (these patients are referred to as patient A, B, C, D, E, F, G, H, K, L). Usually 4 to 5 patients were given each batch of the concentrate being studied. An interval of at least 1 week was observed between treatments, and there were no bleeding episodes at the time of injection, the dose of VIII:C being 25 IU/kg body weight in all cases. Blood samples were collected in citrate (3.8%) immediately before, and 5 and 30 minutes, 1, 2, 4, 6, 9, 11, 24, 36, and 48 hours after injection. Platelet-poor plasma was prepared and stored at -70°C until assayed. Hematocrit was determined before treatment.

Calculations

The plasma volume was calculated according to Allain et al. (15). The in vivo recovery of VIII:C was calculated in the following way:
In vivo recovery (%) =

$$100 \times \frac{\text{plasma volume (ml) x observed rise in VIII:C (IU/ml)}}{\text{injected volume (ml) x labeled potency (IU/ml)}}$$

The plasma concentrations of VIII:C (log) were plotted against time elapsed since injection. The rate of disappearance was determined by least square regression analysis using ^{e}log potencies of the plasma concentrations.

RESULTS AND COMMENTS

In vitro studies

The analytical data for the various factor VIII concentrates are given in Table 2. The low purity concentrates (AHF-Kabi and the cryoprecipitates from Laboratorios Grifols and the Finnisch Red Cross) had the lowest concentrations of VIII:C as assayed by one-stage assay, the values ranging between 2.7 and 7 IU/ml. The concentrates of intermediate purity (Criostat IP and AHF IP, Finish Red Cross) had VIII:C values about 25 IU/ml. The majority of the concentrates were of the high purity, and they had VIII:C values ranging from 25 to 50 IU/ml according to the one-stage assay. DDAVP Octonativ had the highest concentration of VIII:C, namely 100 IU/ml. The VIII:C values obtained with the new chromogenic substrate assay for VIII:C agreed well with those obtained using the one-stage assay. Though our VIII:C estimates were largely in agreement with values given by the manufacturers, there were some exceptions.

With the exception of Factorate, all the concentrates had higher concentrations of factor VIII clotting antigen (VIII:CAg) than of VIII:C indicating inactivation of the clotting activity of factor VIII during the preparation.

The specific activity (IU VIII:C/mg protein) varied considerably from one concentrate to another, even between different batches, being highest in DDAVP Octonativ, Factorate and some batches of Kryobulin and Profilate (~3 IU/mg protein), and lowest in cryoprecipitate and fraction I-0 (~0.2 IU/mg protein). Hemofil T, heat treated in dry state, showed the same specific activity as conventional Hemofil, and the same concentration of VIII:CAg, indicating that the heat treatment procedure in dry state does not cause any further denaturation of the factor VIII clotting component. On the other hand, Profilate HS, heat treated in solution, not only had a considerably lower specific activity than unheated Profilate, but also an VIII:CAg content about three times higher than the conventional concentrate. These results show that the biological activity of factor VIII had been considerably reduced during heating of the product in solution.

It is clear that all types of concentrates contained large amounts of factor VIII/von Willebrand factor — i.e., factor VIII related antigen (VIII:Ag). It is now well known that the von Willebrand factor exists in plasma as a series of multimers ranging in size from approximately 800,000 daltons to over 14×10^6 (16,17). A distinction is usually made between low, intermediate and high molecular weight multimers, and it is now known that only the high molecular weight multimers have von Willebrand factor activity — i.e., the capacity to promote platelet adhesion to subendothelium and maintain normal bleeding time (17,18,19). Patients with variant type II von Willebrand's disease lack the largest multimers of the factor VIII/von Willebrand factor (13,20). Plasma from patients with type II von Willebrand's disease had been found to have normal or almost normal concentrations of VIIIR:Ag (von Willebrand factor) when measured by electroimmunoassay (EIA), but much lower values and non-parallel dose response curves, when measured by immunoradiometric assay (IRMA) (21,22). The discrepancy in results between EIA and IRMA in variant II von Willebrand's disease is believed to be a manifestation of an abnormal molecule.

Values for the VIIIR:Ag concentration in AHF-Kabi (fraction I-0) were much the same whether measured with EIA or IRMA, as was the case with the cryoprecipitates (Table 2). All the intermediate and high purity concentrates had mostly lower concentration of VIIIR:Ag as determined by IRMA (non-parallel dose response curve) than by EIA — i.e., the same pattern as seen in type II von Willebrand's disease patients with a structurally defective von Willebrand factor protein. It should be pointed out that the heat treated Profilate had an extremely high VIIIR:Ag concentration, which is consistent with a marked inactivation of the factor VIII clotting activity during the heating procedure.

Figure 1 shows the multimeric pattern of some of the concentrates studies here. Fraction I-0 (AHF-Kabi) and cryoprecipitate had about the same multimeric composition as normal plasma and thus also contained large multimers. Factorate and Profilate HS had no large multimers and only small amounts of intermediate multimers, especially in the case of Profilate HS, where the pre-dominant bands were of the low molecular weight type. Hemofil and Octonativ also lacked the high molecular weight multimers, but had intermediate and low molecular weight multimers. The results of multimeric sizing of the other concentrates are given in Table 2. From earlier studies it is known that the high purity concentrates, now shown to lack the large multimers, are not capable of correcting the prolonged bleeding time and the hemostatic defect in von Willebrand's disease (23-28). It is also known that cryoprecipitate and fraction I-0, both of which have a normal multimeric pattern, do correct the defect in von Willebrand's disease (25,28-30). It is noteworthy that Thorell and Blombäck (31) recently reported the preparation of two high purity concentrates (specific

Table 2. The in vitro properties of the various concentrates (mean values; the number of batches tested are given in Table I)

	VIII:C I.U./ml		VIII:CAg u/ml	VIIIR:Ag U/ml		VIIIR:RCF u/ml	Fib. mg/I.U. VIII:C	Spec.act. VIII:C I.U./mg prot.	Multimeric sizing
	one-stage assay	chromo-genic assay		EIA	IRMA				
Normal plasma	1	1	1	1	1	1	2-4		All multimers
AHF-Kabi	2.7	2.9	4.6	8	10	4.7	6.1	0.2	-"-
DDAVP-AHF-Kabi	4.5	-	11.3	9	15	-	2.9	0.3	
Octonativ, Kabi	49	55	65	110	59*	45	0.20	2.2	Largest absent
DDAVP Octonativ, Kabi	99	110	219	208	163*	60	0.15	2.8	-"-
Hemofil, Hyland	33	38	43	63	73*	26	0.27	1.6	-"-
Hemofil T, Hyland	35	27	43	82	58*	28	0.28	1.5	-"-
Factorate, Armour	40	36	34	118	23*	8	0.17	3.5	-"-
Kryobulin, Immuno	48	55	119	155	114	50	0.03	2.4	
Profilate, Alpha	24	24	35	50	42*	26	0.6	1.6	-"-
Profilate HS, Alpha	46	41	53	176	36*	14	0.19	2.2	-"-
Criostat Grifols SA	34	33	156	270	260*	-	0.56	0.9	-"-
Criostat IP Grifols SA	28	25	39	110	32-68*	-	0.08	1.8	-"-
Crioprecipitado Grifols SA	28	28	52	164	47*	8	0.34	0.8	-"-
	6	5	11	13	21	8	4.8	0.16	All multimers
Kryo AHG Finnish Red Cross I	6.8	7.0	8.0	7.8	17	11	2.4	0.2	-"-
AHF IP Finnish Red Cross II	22	21	29	39	18*	22	0.8	0.7	Largest absent

*) non-parallel dose response curves

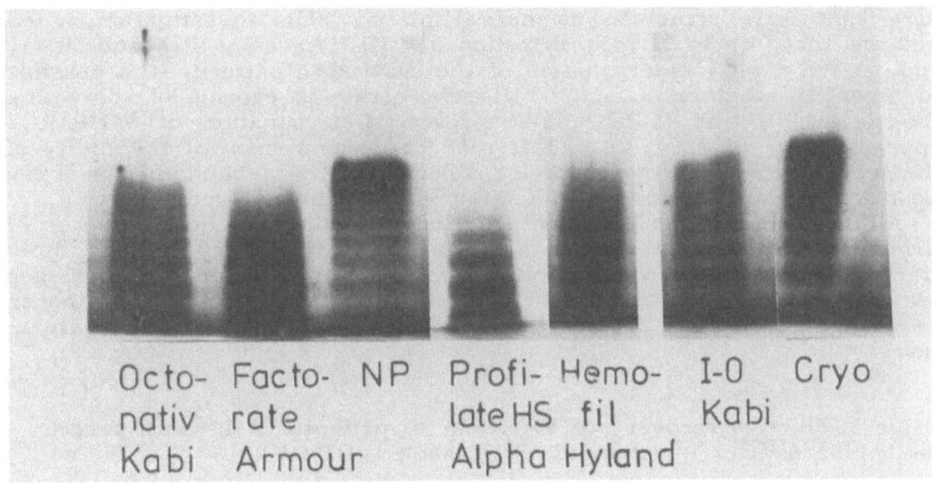

Figure 1. SDS electrophoresis in 1.6% agarose of VIIIR:Ag in a
discontinuous pH buffer system. Samples (from the left):
Octonativ (Kabi), Factorate (Armour), normal plasma, Profilate
HS (Alpha, Hemofil (Hyland), fraction I-0 (AHF-Kabi) and
cryoprecipitate.

activity 2.5 and 7.6 IU VIII:C/mg protein), which were able to correct
the prolonged bleeding time in severe von Willebrand's disease and were
found to have a normal multimeric pattern. This appears to be the only
available high purity concentrate containing functional von Willebrand
factor. They used cryoprecipitate as starting material and removed
fibrinogen by adding glycine (2.0 M), factor VIII being precipitated by
the addition of solid sodium chloride.

Several workers have now shown that determination of ristocetin
cofactor activity (VIIIR:RCF) fails to reflect the bleeding time corrective
properties of the factor VIII/von Willebrand factor in factor VIII concentrates (23-26,32). We found that, with the exception of the cryoprecipitates, the values for VIIIR:RCF in the concentrates were much
lower than those for VIIIR:Ag as determined by EIA, and roughly
corresponded to those for VIII:C (Table 2). Similar results have been
reported by Allain et al (15) and by Barrowcliffe et al (33).

The most physiologically relevant in vitro test of the von Willebrand
factor activity appears to be factor VIII/von Willebrand factor mediated
adhesion of platelets to subendothelium (34). Sixma et al (35) have
studied platelet adherence to the subendothelium of human umbilical
arteries in an annular perfusion chamber in the presence of various
factor VIII concentrates. They found that cryoprecipitate and fraction
I-0 were capable of promoting platelet adhesion, while high purity
factor VIII concentrates were not.

From the above mentioned studies of factor VIII/von Willebrand factor
in different factor VIII concentrates, it seems clear that, to be able to
correct the bleeding time and normalize the hemostatic defect, the

factor VIII related protein must be present in a native form with the same multimeric structure as normal plasma. The investigations cited indicate that, by in vitro examination of VIIIR:Ag using EIA and IRMA, and, above all, by determination of the multimeric pattern, it is possible to ascertain whether a factor VIII concentrate is capable of correcting the defect in von Willebrand's disease. Determination of VIIIR:RCF appears to be of no value in this respect. Measurement of the ability of the concentrate to promote platelet adhesion to the subendothelium is the most sophisticated method of detecting von Willebrand factor activity.

All the concentrates contain fibrinogen (Table 2). Some batches of Kryobulin and Croistat-Grifols had the lowest fibrinogen content. Both fraction I-0 and the cryoprecipitates have a high content of fibrinogen per unit VIII:C, which raises the question of whether the fibrinogen may not in some way protect factor VIII related protein from denaturation.

Table 3. In vivo recovery of VIII:C in 10 patients (A-L) with severe hemophilia A after injection of 25 IU labeled VIII:C/kg.

	A	B	C	D	E	F	G	H	K	L	Mean
					PATIENTS						
AHF- Kabi	79				67		68		69	-	71
Octonativ			78	121		89	90	105			97
DDAVP Octonativ			75	104		96	99	126			100
Hemofil			67		86	74					76
Hemofil T			65		78	82	100				81
Profilate	78	79	53	64							69
Profilate HS	110	79	80	84							88

Table 4. Half-life (h) of VIII:C in 10 patients (A-L) with severe hemophilia A after injection of 25 IU labeled VIII:C/kg.

	A	B	C	D	E	F	G	H	K	L	Mean
					PATIENTS						
AHF-Kabi	18		-	-	15		17		17	-	17
Octonativ			17	7		15	12	9			12
DDAVP Octonativ			16	9		14	10	12			12
Hemofil			14		10	15					13
Hemofil T			15		10	13	15				13
Profilate	16	15	20	10							15
Profilate HS	16	14	18	7							14

The concentrates prepared from DDAVP plasma contained about twice as much VIII:C and VIIIR:Ag as did corresponding control fractions, but otherwise no differences in the in vitro properties were seen.

In vivo studies

In our in vivo studies, the same group of patients with hemophilia A were given the same number of units of factor VIII per kg body weight (25 IU labeled VIII:C/kg). In vivo recovery was calculated from the increase in VIII:C observed 5 min after injection, and was about the same for all the preparations and varied between 65 and 100% (Table 3). The peak of circulating VIII:C was regularly observed in the samples taken immediately after the infusion; this is in contrast to the findings of some workers (15,36) who have reported a higher VIII:C recovery in samples drawn one hour after injection.

The half-life was estimated from observations during the late phase of clearance, between 5 and 48 hours after injection (Table 4). All the high purity concentrates had about the same half-life varying between 10-17 hours. In most published reports (15,25,36-39) the half-life for more purified concentrates has been found to vary between 5-20 hours with a mean of about 12 hours. AHF-Kabi (fraction I-0) had a somewhat longer half-life, 15-18 hours, which is in agreement with our earlier studies (6,25) (fig. 2). Other in vivo studies have also indicated a relatively longer biological half-life of VIII:C in less purified material such as plasma and cryoprecipitates (40-43). DDAVP Octonativ had the same half-life as ordinary Octonativ, which has earlier been shown by Mikaelsson et al (39). Heat treated Hemofil and heat treated Profilate (fig. 3) had the same half-life as the concentrates prepared in conventional way. In most of the survival studies VIII:C was also assessed by the chromogenic VIII:C assay. These values agreed extremely well with those obtained by the one-stage assay (figs. 2,3).

Our earlier in vivo studies (25,27,28) have clearly shown that only fraction I-0 and cryoprecipitate are able to correct the prolonged bleeding in patients with severe von Willebrand's disease.

CONCLUDING REMARKS

Several differences in the in vitro properties were found in this study of 3 low purity concentrates (fraction I-0 and freeze-dried cryoprecipitates), 2 intermediate concentrates and 6 commercial high purity concentrates, two heat treated concentrates and 2 concentrates prepared from DDAVP stimulated blood donors.

VIII:C values obtained from a chromogenic substrate assay showed good correlation with those obtained by one-stage assay. The specific activity (IU VIII:C/mg protein) varied considerably from one concentrate to another, even between different batches, being highest in DDAVP Octonativ, Factorate and some batches of Kryobulin and Profilate (3 IU/mg protein) and lowest in cryoprecipitate and fraction I-0 (0.2 IU/mg protein). Heat treated Hemofil T, had the same specific activity as non-heated Hemofil while heat treated Profilate had lower specific activity than non-heated Profilate. With the exception of Factorate, all preparations had higher concentrations of VIII:CAg than of VIII:C, indicating inactivation of the biological activity of VIII:C during preparation.

Studies of the factor VIII/von Willebrand factor showed that all the concentrates contain considerable amounts of VIIIR:Ag, as measured by electroimmunoassay. When measured immunoradiometrically, the values for VIIIR:Ag concentrations were lower, both for intermediate and high purity concentrates, than when measured with an electroimmunoassay, and the dose response curves were non-parallel. Multimeric sizing demonstrated that all the intermediate and high purity concentrates lacked the high molecular weight multimers. AHF-Kabi (fraction I-0) and the cryoprecipitates, the only preparations capable of correcting the bleeding defect in patients with von Willebrand's disease, were found to have the same multimeric pattern as normal plasma, and the values for their VIIIR:Ag concentrations did not vary appreciably from those obtained with an IRMA. Based on these in vitro techniques, it seems possible to predict which preparations will be succesful in treating patients with von Willebrand's disease, while no such conclusions can be drawn from VIIIR:RCF analysis.

The concentrates prepared from DDAVP plasma contained at least twice as much VIII:C and VIIIR:Ag as corresponding control fractions, but otherwise no differences in its in vitro properties were seen.

In the in vivo studies, the recovery of VIII:C was about the same for all the preparations (65-100%). The half-life was about the same for all the high purity concentrates, varying between 10 and 17 h, though AHF-Kabi (fraction I-0) had a somewhat longer half-life, 15-18 h. Only fraction I-0 and the cryoprecipitates are able to correct the prolonged bleeding time in patients with severe vWD.

The feasibility of monitoring hemophilia therapy by means of the chromogenic substrate assay was clearly demonstrated.

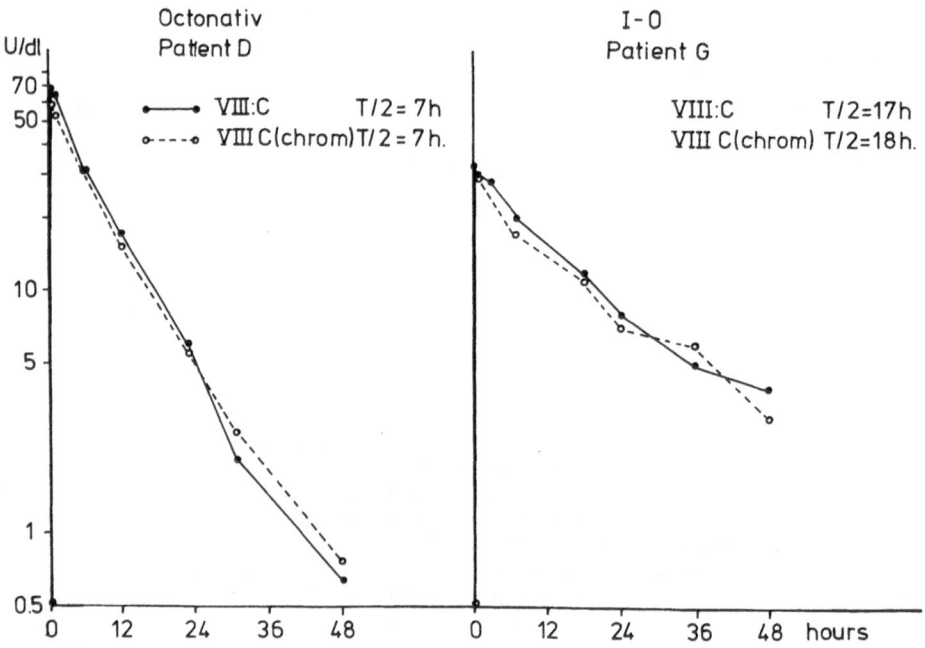

Figure 2. In vivo disappearance curves in patient D after injection of Octonativ and in patient G after injection of fraction I-O (AHF-Kabi). The dose was 25 IU/kg body weight. VIII:C was assessed by both the one-stage clotting method and the chromogenic substrage method.

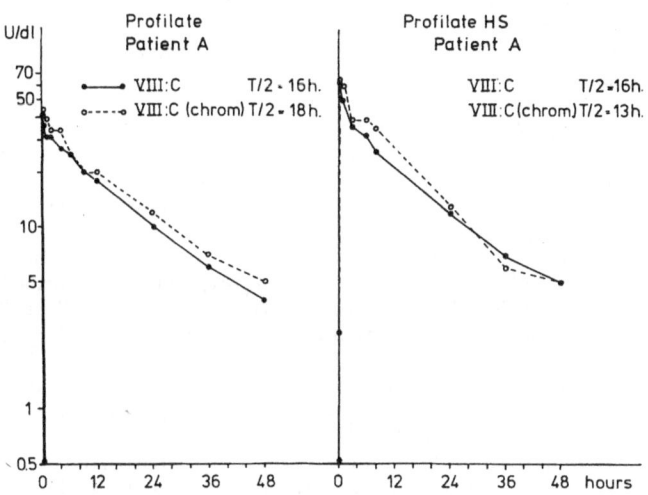

Figure 3. In vivo disappearance curves in patient A after injection of Profilate and heat treated Profilate (Profilate HS). The dose was 25 IU/ kg body weight. VIII:C was assessed by both the one-stage clotting method and the chromogenic substrate method.

ACKNOWLEDGEMENT

The investigation was supported by grants from the Swedish Medical Research Council (00087).
Some of the results have been published earlier (Nilsson IM, Borge L, Gunnarsson M, Kristofferson AC: Factor VIII related activities in concentrates: Scand J Haematol 1984;33(suppl.41):157-72.

REFERENCES

1. Blombäck B, Blombäck M. Purification of human and bovine fibrinogen. Arkiv Kemi 1956;20:415-43.
2. Nilsson IM, Blombäck M, Ramgren O. Haemophilia in Sweden. VI. Treatment of haemophilia A with the human antihaemophilic factor preparation (fraction I-0). Acta Med Scand 1962;379:61-110.
3. Mikaelsson M, Nilsson IM, Vilhardt H, Wiechel B. Factor VIII concentrate prepared from blood donors stimulated by intranasal administration of a vasopressin analogue. Transfusion 1982;22: 229-33.
4. Nilsson IM, Blombäck M, von Francken I. On an inherited autosomal hemorrhagic diathesis with antihemophilic globulin (AHG) deficiency and prolonged bleeding time. Acta Med Scand 1957;159:35-57.
5. Nilsson IM. Haemorrhagic and thrombotic diseased. John Wiley & Sons, London, 1974.

6. Nilsson IM, Kirkwood TBL, Barrowcliffe TW. In vivo recovery of factor VIII: A comparison of one-stage and two stage assay methods. Thrombos Haemostas 1979;42:1230-9.

7. Rosén S. Assay of Factor VIII:C with a chromogenic substrate. Scand J Haematol 1984;40:139-45.

8. Holmberg L, Borge L, Ljung R, Nilsson IM. Measurement of anti-haemophilic factor A antigen (VIII:CAg) with a solid phase immuno-radiometric method based on homologous non-haemophilic antibodies. Scand J Haematol 1979;23:17-24.

9. Holmberg L, Nilsson IM. Genetic variants of von Willebrand's disease. Br Med J 1972;3:317-20.

10. Ruggeri ZM, Mannucci PM, Jeffcoate SL, Ingram GIC. Immunoradio-metric assay of factor VIII related antigen, with observations in 32 patients with von Willebrand's disease. Br J Haematol 1976;33:221-32.

11. Holmberg L, Ljung R. Purification of F VIII:C by antigen antibody chromatography. Thromb Res 1978;12:667-75.

12. Zuzel M, Nilsson IM, Åberg M. A method for measuring plasma ristocetin cofactor activity. Normal distribution and stability during storage. Thromb Res 1978;12:745-54.

13. Ruggeri ZM, Zimmerman TS. The complex multimeric composition of factor VIII/von Willebrand factor. Blood 1981;57:1140-4.

14. Nilsson IM, Olow B. Determination of fibrinogen and fibrinogenolytic activity. Thromb Diath Haemorrh 1962;8:297-310.

15. Allain JP, Verroust F, Soulier JP. In vitro and in vivo characteriza-tion of factor VIII preparations. Vox Sang 1980;38:68-80.

16. Hoyer LW, Shainoff JR. Factor VIII-related protein circulates in normal human plasma as high molecular weight multimers. Blood 1980;55:1056-9.

17. Ruggeri ZM, Zimmerman TS. Variant von Willebrand's disease: characterization of two subtypes by analysis of multimeric composition of factor VIII/ von Willebrand factor in plasma and platelets. J Clin Invest 1980;65:1318-25.

18. Counts RB, Paskell SL, Elgee SK. Disulfide bonds and the quaternary structure of factor VIII/von Willebrand factor. J Clin Invest 1978;62:702-9.

19. Sakariassen KS, Bolhuis PA, Sixma JJ. Human blood platelet adhesion to artery subendothelium is mediated by factor VIII/von Willebrand factor bound to the subendothelium. Nature 1979;279:636-8.

20. Ruggeri ZM, Nilsson IM, Lombardi R, Holmberg L, Zimmerman TS. Aberrant multimeric structure of von Willebrand factor in a new variant of von Willebrand's disease (type IIC). J Clin Invest 1982;70:1124-7.

21. Peake IR, Bloom AL. Abnormal factor VIII related antigen (FVIIIRAG) in von Willebrand's disease (vWD): Decreased precipitation by a con-canavalin A. Thrombos Haemostas 1977;37:361-2.

22. Nilsson IM, Peake IR, Bloom AL, Meyer D, Veltkamp JJ, Green D. Report of the Working Party on factor VIII related antigens. Thrombos Haemostas 1980;43:167-8.

23. Blatt PM, Brinkhous KM, Culp HR, Krauss JS, Roberts HR. Anti-hemophilic factor concentrate therapy in von Willebrand disease. Dissociation of bleeding-time factor and ristocetin-cofactor activities. J Am Med Ass 1976;236:2770-2.

24. Green D, Potter EV. Failure of AHF concentrate to control bleeding in von Willebrand's disease. Am J Med 1976;60:357-61.

25. Nilsson IM, Hedner U. Characteristics of various factor VIII con-centrates used in treatment of haemophilia A. Br J Haematol 1977;37:543-57.

26. Weinstein M, Deykin D. Comparison of factor VIII-related von Willebrand factor proteins prepared from human cryoprecipitate and factor VIII concentrate. Blood 1979;53:1095-1105.
27. Nilsson IM, Holmberg L. von Willebrand's disease today. Clin Haematol 1979;8147-68.
28. Nilsson IM von Willebrand's disease from 1926-1983. Scand J Haematol 1984;suppl 40)33:21-43.
29. Bennett E, Dormandy K. Pool's cryoprecipitate and exhausted plasma in the treatment of von Willebrand's disease and factor XI-deficiency. Lancet 1966;ii:731-2.
30. Perkins HA. Correction of the hemostatic defects in von Willebrand's disease. Blood 1967;30:375-80.
31. Thorell L, Blombäck B. Purification of the factor VIII complex. Thromb Res 1984;35:431-50.
32. Mannucci PM, Pareti FI, Holmberg L, Nilsson IM, Ruggeri ZM. Studies on the prolonged bleeding time in von Willebrand's disease. J Lab Clin Med 1976;88:662-71.
33. Barrowcliffe TW, Kemball-Cook G, Morris G, Holt JC, Furlong RA, Peake IR. Factor VIII-related activities in therapeutic concentrates. J Lab Clin Med 1981;97:429-38.
34. Baumgartner HR, Tschopp TB, Mayer D. Shear rate dependent inhibition of platelet adhesion and aggregation on collagenous surfaces by antibodies to human factor VIII/von Willebrand factor. Br J Haematol 1980;44:127-39.
35. Sixma JJ, Sakariassen KS, Beeser-Visser NG, Ottenhof-Rovers M, Bolhuis PA. Adhesion of platelets to human artery subendothelium: Effect of factor VIII − von Willebrand factor of various multimeric composition. Blood 1984;63:128-40.
36. Allain JP. Principles of in vivo recovery and survival studies. Scand J Haematol 1984;33(suppl 40):123-30.
37. Brinkhous KM, Shanbrom E, Roberts HR, Webster WP, Fekete L, Wagener RH. A new high potency glycine-precipitated antihemophilic factor (AHF) concentrate: Treatment of classical hemophilia and hemophilia with inhibitors. J Am Med Ass 1968,250:613-7.
38. Schimpf K, Scherenberg R. Recovery and survival of factor VIII concentrates. Proc IX cong WF Haemophilia, Istanbul, Aug 20-22. 1974.
39. Mikaelsson M, Nilsson IM, Cedergren B, Jonsson S, Rydberg L, Wiechel B. The use of Desmopressin (DDAVP) in the preparation of improved factor VIII concentrates. Scand J Haematol 1984;33 (suppl 40):93-101.
40. Abildgaard CF, Simone JV, Corrigan JJ et al. Treatment of hemophilia with glycine-precipitated factor VIII. N Engl J Med 1966;275:471-5.
41. Pool JG, Shannon AE. Production of high-potency concentrates of antihaemophilic globulin in a closed-bag system. N Engl J Med 1965;273:1443-7.
42. Verstraete M, Lust A, Vermylen J. In vitro and in vivo recovery of cryoprecipitated factor VIII. Proc 5th cong WF haemophilia, Montreal, 1968.
43. Allain JP, Etude de l'activité "in vivo" du Facteur VIII ou du Facteur IX après injection de différents concentrés: applications pratiques. Nouv Rev Franç Hématol 1972;12:241-9.

CLINICAL USE OF POLYELECTROLYTE-FRACTIONATED PORCINE FACTOR VIII

P.B.A Kernoff

There is no shortage of animal plasma and, in several species, plasma factor VIII levels are higher than they are in man — in the case of pigs, about five times higher (1). These advantages were recognised by Dr. Ethel Bidwell and her colleagues, who prepared the first animal factor VIII concentrates for intravenous human therapeutic use in the early 1950's (2).

The early animal factor VIII concentrates were clearly capable of stopping and preventing bleeding in hemophiliacs but they did have major disadvantages, particularly as regards their high risk of adverse effects. Because of these problems, and the increasing availability of human concentrates, they fell into disuse from the mid 1960's.

The porcine factor VIII concentrate whose clinical use will be described, called Hyate:C by its manufacturers Speywood Laboratories, differs in some fundamental respects from these early conventionally-prepared porcine concentrates, not least in its method of fractionation using ethylene maleic anhydride polyelectrolytes (PEs) (3).

Table 1. Comparative product characteristics of conventional and PE-fractionated porcine VIII concentrates (representative batches). VIII:C was assayed using a human concentrate standard. VIII:RAg and PAF were assayed using a porcine plasma standard.

	Conventional	PE
VIII:C U/ml	12	25
VIII:RAg U/ml	27	2
PAF U/ml	20	1
Protein mg/ml	25	1
Specific Activity VIII:C U/mg protein	0.5	25
Solution time	30 mins	1 min

Some of these differences are shown in Table 1. In particular, PE porcine VIII is of much higher purity, contains minimal concentrations of VIII:RAg and its associated biological activity (platelet aggregating factor, PAF), and dissolves almost instantaneously. As regards purity, it should be noted that the specific activity of PE porcine VIII is at least 5-10 times higher than the purest human factor VIII concentrates currently available for therapeutic use.

Although the early porcine factor VIII concentrates were used to treat patients both with and without inhibitors, the present use of the product is largely confined to those in the former group. The rationale of use in these patients is that inhibitors in hemophilic plasmas almost invariably react less strongly with porcine factor VIII than they do with human factor VIII. Therefore, use of porcine VIII allows one to extend the number of patients and bleeding episodes which can be managed successfully with factor VIII, without having to resort to PCCs or APCCs.

Table 2. Advantages of PE porcine VIII.

— few plasma supply problems
— high porcine plasma VIII level
— reduced reactivity of porcine VIII with most inhibitors
— high purity of product
— known active constituent, so conventional methods of control
— lesser or absent risk of hepatitis and other human viral transmission
— most effective therapy in selected patients
— cost/benefit advantages in selected patients

In patients who have never previously been exposed to animal concentrates, cross-reactivity against porcine VIII averages about 25% of that towards human VIII, but can differ very much between patients — in our studies, from nil to 80%. As might be expected, and as we have found in clinical practice, both post-infusion factor VIII recovery and clinical response are inversely related to pre-treatment inhibitor levels to porcine VIII — in other words, the higher the inhibitor level, the less good the response. To some extent, the level of inhibitors to porcine VIII can be predicted from knowledge of the anti-human level, which simplifies assessment (4,5). Because of all these relationships, conventional laboratory methods can be used both to guide patient selection and control dosage.

One additional possible advantage of porcine VIII, which is increasingly perceived by our patients, is the probable lesser or absent risk of contamination with human hepatitis and other viruses, such as the putative AIDS agent. This is both because of the nature of the source plasma and the disinfecting potential of polyelectrolyte fractionation (6).

We have used PE porcine VIII to treat patients with inhibitors since 1980. Over this four year period, more than 1,500 infusions have been given to ten patients to treat both major and minor bleeding episodes, to provide prophylaxis by home therapy, and to cover elective surgery. Repeated and porlonged courses of treatment have been given to some patients without loss of clinical or laboratory efficacy. In others, however, repeated dosing may be accompanied by diminishing effect, and the product is not without its disadvantages (Table 3).

Table 3. Disadvantages of PE porcine VIII.

— can cause anamnestic rise in inhibitor level in susceptible patients
— not usually effective at high inhibitor levels (>50-100 B.U.)
— ? limitation on number/duration of courses of therapy: 'resistance'
— occasional adverse effects: reactions, thrombocytopenia
— can be expensive in high dosage
— must be stored in freezer

One problem, which in my view has been somewhat overstated, is its potential, like human factor VIII, to cause anamnestic rises in inhibitor levels in susceptible patients. It needs to be remembered that the primary objective of treatment is usually to stop or prevent bleeding, rather than trying to avoid a rise in inhibitor levels. Where circulating levels of factor VIII can be achieved after infusion of therapeutic product, there is little disagreement that clinical responses after either porcine or human factor VIII, are superior to those generally obtainable using PCCs or APCCs. Also, the occurrence and magnitude of an anamnestic response after factor VIII is by no means always predictable, even in patients categorised as 'high responders'. However, because of this problem with anamnestic responses, our general policy has shifted over the last two years, in most patients at least, towards less frequent use of porcine VIII in mild bleeding episodes. We currently use 'cold' factor IX concentrate for such events in high responding patients, trading therapeutic efficacy for a lesser chance of invoking an anamnestic response.

A second problem with porcine VIII is that it is not very effective at high inhibitor levels. Most patients with less than about 50 Bethesda units to human factor VIII at the time of treatment respond favourably to porcine VIII, especially with repeated dosing, and some patients with particularly low cross-reactivity show good clinical responses at up to 100 B.U. Above 100 B.U., favourable clinical responses are less likely unless massive doses are used. The highest dose being used was 500 U/kg.

So far as the well-documented adverse effects of the early porcine VIII concentrates are concerned — namely, transfusion reaction and acute thrombocytopenia — the polyelectrolyte-fractionated product seems to be much safer. However, we have very occasionally seen these problems and recommend a high level of surveillance. In high dosage, porcine VIII can be expensive and the company is going to have to look carefully at their pricing policy if cost is not going to limit therapeutic applicability.

Although our experience with porcine VIII and surgery is not large (Table 4), we have not seen problems with bleeding. One patient, a low responder, has had two major elective orthopaedic procedures without complications, and is delighted with the results. He is now been

Table 4. Elective surgery and PE porcine VIII.

	Pre-surgery inhibitor level to human VIII	Surgery
Patient 1 (low responder)	5 B.U.	Ulnar nerve decompression
	3 B.U.	Knee joint replacement
Patient 2 (high responder)	19 B.U.	Nasal polypectomy
Patient 3 (high responder)	97 B.U.	Hemorrhoid injection
Patient 4 (non-inhibitor)	NIL	Anterior resection of carcinoma of rectum

on alternate day self-administered prophylaxis with porcine VIII for three years. In two other patients, both high responders, porcine VIII alone has provided sufficient length of cover for two less major surgical procedures, although anamnestic responses occurred at about a week post-operatively. In a fourth patient, a man with mild hemophilia and without inhibitors (basal factor VIII 12 U/dl), porcine VIII was used to cover major abdominal surgery in an attempt to avoid post-transfusion hepatitis. Decreasing laboratory responses from day 5 suggested the development of an inhibitor, which reached a peak of 3 B.U. to porcine VIII on day 10.

No cross-reaction with human factor VIII was demonstrable, and a change to human factor VIII was followed by restoration of normal laboratory responses, and maintenance of clinical control. Unfortunately, but perhaps not unexpectedly, non-A non-B hepatitis occurred six weeks after starting therapy with human factor VIII. In a similar non-inhibitor patient, treated by Dr. Wensley and his colleagues in Manchester, surgical cover with porcine VIII could be limited to a few days duration, and posttransfusion hepatitis did not occur (7).

Anyone who has had to take responsibility for the management of hemophiliacs with inhibitors would agree that there is no one answer to treatment, or any one ideal therapeutic product. To get the best clinical results, treatment has to be carefully tailored to the individual patient and the individual bleeding episode. Because of the inherently serious nature of the disorder, risks often have to be taken with potentially dangerous therapeutic materials, and many factors may influence the choice of such products (Table 5). In my view, the two most important factors are the severity of the clinical problem, and the patient's likely or measured inhibitor levels at the time therapy is needed. Our current strategy for the treatment of inhibitors patients, and the use of porcine VIII, are mainly based on these two factors (Table 6). This strategy has evolved over more than four years experience with porcine VIII, and after many helpful discussions of the issues with colleagues in other institutions.

Table 5. Factors influencing selection of therapeutic product for treatment of inhibitor patients.

— inhibitor level at time of treatment
— severity of bleed/clinical problem
— patients' previous responses
— cross-reactivity of inhibitor against porcine VIII
— likelihood of anamnestic rise in anti-VIII level
— cost
— kinetic characteristics of inhibitor
— transmissible disease/adverse effects

Table 6. Policy for initial management.

Pre-treatment inhibitor level to human VIII	First choice therapeutic product
<5 B.U.	— mild bleeds/low responders: human VIII 20-50 U/kg — mild bleeds/high responders: PCC 50 U/kg — severe bleeds: porcine VIII 20-50 U/kg
5-50 B.U.	— mild bleeds: PCC 50 U/kg — severe bleeds: porcine VIII 50-100 U/kg
>50 B.U.	— PCC 50 U/kg or porcine VIII 100 U/kg if severe bleed and low cross-reactivity (anti-porcine VIII <15 B.U.)

In patients with low level inhibitors who are known low responders, we generally use human factor VIII for mild bleeding, and porcine VIII for more serious episodes. High responding patients who have inhibitor levels less than about 50 B.U. are usually treated with 'cold' factor IX concentrate for mild bleeds, both to limit the chances of anamnesis and to limit expenditure — factor IX concentrate in the UK is free at the point of consumption. For more serious bleeding, when effective hemostatic control becomes the highest priority, these patients are treated with porcine VIII under full laboratory control. In the most difficult group of patients, those with very high level inhibitors, treatment is generally started with factor IX concentrate while the inhibitory activity to porcine factor VIII is determined by direct assay. If the level of anti-porcine VIII is less than about 15 B.U., and the bleed is serious, porcine factor VIII in high dosage is given. If the level of anti-porcine VIII is higher, and factor IX concentrate seems insufficiently effective, one of the two commercial APCCs is considered. Sometimes, of course, none of these measures works.

Polyelectrolyte-fractionated porcine factor VIII is not the complete answer to the problem of management of hemophiliacs with inhibitors, but I am convinced that it does represent a genuine advance. Used carefully in properly selected patients, and to optimum dosage, it is a valuable addition to our therapeutic options.

REFERENCES

1. Bennett B, Ratnoff WD: Immunologic relationships of antihemophilic factor of different species detected by specific human and rabbit antibodies. Proc Soc Biol Med 1973;143:701-6.
2. Bidwell E: The purification of antihaemophilic globulin from animal plasma. Br J Haematol 1955;1:386-9.
3. Middleton S: Polyelectrolytes and preparation of factor VIIIC. In: Forbes CD, Lowe GDO, eds. Unresolved problems in haemophilia. Lancaster. MTP Press, 1982:109-20.

4. Kernoff PBA, Thomas ND, Lilley PA, Matthews KB, Goldman E, Tuddenham EGD: Clinical experience with polyelectrolyte-fractionated porcine factor VIII concentrate in the treatment of hemophiliacs with antibodies to factor VIII. Blood 1984;63:31-41.
5. Kernof PBA: Porcine factor VIII: preparation and use in treatment of inhibitor patients. In: Hoyer LW, ed. Factor VIII inhibitors. New York, Alan R. Liss 1984:207-24.
6. Galpin SA, Karayiannis P, Middleton SM, Thomas HC: The removal of hepatitis B virus from factor VIII concentrates by fractionation on ethylene maleic anhydride polyelectrolyte. J Med Virol: 1984; 14:229-33.
7. Wensley RT, Delamore IW, Burn AM, Cottrell S, Maugham L: The use of porcine factor VIII concentrate to cover major surgery in a mildly affected haemophiliac. Proc XVI Cong Wrld Fed Hemophilia 1984:19 (Abstr).

FACTOR VIII:C ASSAY STANDARDISATION

P.C. Das, P.H.M.J. Thijssen, R.L. McShine, C.Th. Smit Sibinga

Plasma Factor VIII is a complex molecule. Not only is it labile but it also has different functional activities, one being the clotting activity. For the treatment of hemophilia A patients, therapeutic products containing Factor VIII:C are being produced by Blood Banks and industry. For providing accurate product labels for the different therapeutic materials standardised assay is of considerable importance. Austen et al. (1) have found 20% overlabelling and Kasper (2) has warned clinicians to be aware that plasma levels of Factor VIII after infusion might be lower than they would predict from the unitage on the label. The development of well studied local standards calibrated against well known international materials is of considerable importance in this matter (3). While gathering certain knowledge and expertise, there is a certain classical path one follows (fig. 1) when generating and studying local standards, to be linked to well established international materials (4). The aim of this report is to analyse our experience on factor VIII determination, its variations and error within our own laboratory. Secondly, we report on the development of a local plasma standard, and a local concentrate standard.

Factor VIII has been assayed in our laboratory by the one stage method (aPTT) using commercial kits. Dilutions of tests and standards were in replicates. It was made sure that clotting times of known and test samples overlapped, the dose response curves were linear, and their drifts checked and minimised. It should be emphasized that the parallelism of the curve is important. However, for calculation one needs a special mathematical program and this has not yet been established in our laboratory. The initial study was carried out with pooled plasma (20 donors), part of which was freeze-dried and the rest kept frozen (Table 1). In this study a freshly collected normal pool of plasma provided the standard. The study as carried out over a length of time by 2 different observers, suggests that the freeze-dried material behaved more consistently, with less coefficient of variation than the frozen plasma. Since one unit of factor VIII activity is defined as the amount present in 1 ml of fresh citrated plasma, the study allows to visualise the range of factor VIII:C activity to be encountered, based on the local fresh plasma. Thus, the choice fell upon this freeze-dried plasma to be calibrated against the international plasma standard (5). This second phase was very labour intensive, starting in 1983 and continued till 1984. The recent WHO plasma standard (80/511) was obtained from London, its mean potency being 0.73 IU. Against this, our own first plasma standard (L.P.) gave a value of 1.24 IU (Table 2). This incidentally, was the same figure that had been obtained using fresh plasma in our earlier study (Table 1). A reversed order of tests showed 0.73 IU for the WHO material, which is the quoted mean value for this international standard.

Our second and third plasma standards were made. In the initial calibration, the first local standard has been used as the standard, which was however, by this time 4 months old. The figure of 1.2 IU to the second and 1.3 IU to the third local standard, was given temporarily as we suspected these figures to be dubious. On rechecking with the

218

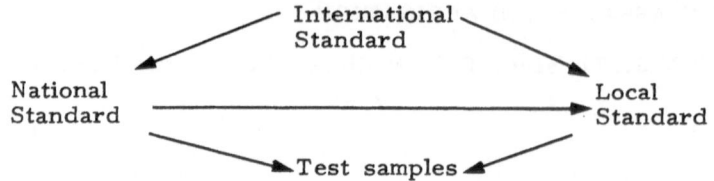

Figure 1. Scheme of factor VIII standardization

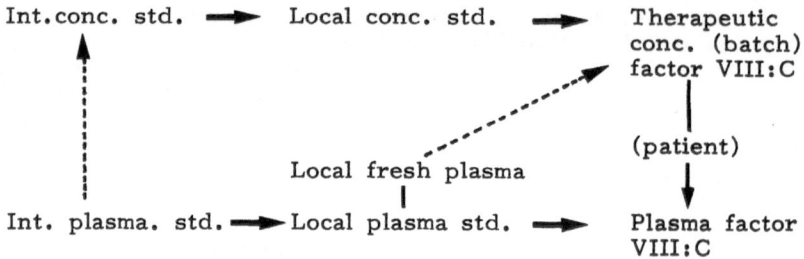

Figure 2. Local scheme for standardization of plasma and concentrate materials — for in vitro and in vivo assessment. Direct link is in unbroken line, and indirect link on broken line.

Table 1. Factor VIII(C) assay on plasma (IU/ml).

Frozen		Freeze dried	
$\bar{x}$:	1.52	$\bar{x}$:	1.24
SD :	0.28	SD :	0.08
CV :	19.0	CV :	6.4

Table 2. Standardization of plasma for factor VIII:C (IU/ml) 11/83, 5/84.

Reference material	Studies and values		
3rd international plasma standard (WHO, 1983)	1st L.P. standard	$\bar{x}$ 1,24	(± 0.05)
1st local plasma standard	2nd local plasma standard	$\bar{x}$ 1,26	(± 0.10)
	3rd local plasma standard	$\bar{x}$ 1,31	(± 0.11)

Table 3. Standardization of plasma factor VIII:C (IU/ml).

Reference material	Studies and values		
international plasma standard		5/84	8/84
(WHO, 1983)	2nd local plasma standard	x̄ 0.78 (± 0.04)	x̄ 0.73 (± 0.03)
	3rd local plasma standard	x̄ 0.97 (± 0.06)	x̄ 0.86 (± 0.06)
	4th local plasma standard		x̄ 0.86 (± 0.02

international plasma standard the figure for the second local standard appeared to be 0.78 IU and for the third plasma standard 0.97 IU (Table 3). This was consistently found between May and early summer of 1984, when the tests were repeated using the international material as the standard.

The current fourth local plasma standard has been calibrated against the international material showing 0.86 IU/ml (Table 3). The explanation for this is not clear, but there is an important lesson to be learned. The freeze-dried material was stored in an ordinary freezer, perhaps -20°C or lower would have been better. The stability of the plasma standard is enhanced when it is buffered before freeze drying (6) and we have not done so. After coupling with the international standard, it should have been "spied" on its behaviour in the time. With reflections we became wiser: We now call the local standard "tiger", and this is being followed, day to day, by materials called "jackal". The tiger moves very quietly, but almost always is being followed by jackals who expect to share the kills. As the tiger moves, one can trace the movements by the regular but intermittent howls of the following jackals.

The third phase of the study relates to the standardisation and development of a local concentrate standard (Table 4). It is well recognised that likes should be measured with likes: Plasma with plasma, concentrates with concentrates. Traditionally, this wisdom has not been adhered to, partly due to local difficulties, but mostly because the definition of factor VIII units is linked to plasma. The local concentrate standard consisted of a freeze dried pool of 6 cryoprecipitates. Against the local plasma standard, the value of the cryoprecipitate was 7.4 IU in March 1984 and 8.4 IU in April 1984. Although the standard deviation was considerable, it should be emphasized that we were becoming little suspicious about the plasma standard as mentioned earlier. Against the international concentrate WHO standard (80/556) obtained from London, the first local cryo standard has scored a value of 8.5 IU. This seems to be excellent, but instead we became worried. Our concern seems to be justified since against the freshly made fourth local plasma standard and against the international plasma standard, the cryoprecipitate seems to contain 4.6 IU, instead of 7-8 IU (Table 4).

The mechanism and cause of this remains unclear, but pragmatically we decided that the first cryoprecipitate was not suitable as local concentrate standard. We developed a second pooled cryoprecipitate. Studies carried out on freeze-dried material during the summer of 1984 did show

Table 4. Standardization of concentrate factor VIII:C (IU/ml): 1st local cryo concentrate.

Reference material	Studies and values		
		3/84	4/84
1st local plasma standard	1st local cryo concentrate	$\bar{x}$ 7.41 (± 1.30)	$\bar{x}$ 8.44 (± 2.10)
Int. conc. standard (WHO, 1983)	1st local cryo concentrate		$\bar{x}$ 8.50 (± 0.30)
		5/84	
Int. plasma standard (WHO, 1983)	1st local cryo concentrate	$\bar{x}$ 4.52	(± 0.70)
4th local plasma standard	1st local cryo concentrate	$\bar{x}$ 4.65	(± 0.63)

Table 5. Standardization of concentrates factor VIII:C (IU/ml): 2nd local concentrate.

Reference material	Studies and values	
		6-8/84
Int. concentrate standard (WHO, 1983)	2nd local cryo concentrate	$\bar{x}$ 5.12 (± 0.39)
Int. plasma standard (WHO, 1983)	2nd local cryo concentrate	$\bar{x}$ 4.35 (± 0,86)

a mean value of 5.1 IU against the international concentrate standard, and 4.4 IU against the international plasma standard (Table 5).

We are much happier with these figures since it appears that with plasma a concentrate gives relatively low values, while higher values are generally obtained against a concentrate standard (7). However, the local standard has been sent to London to obtain a second opinion. It is well recognised that the measured values of well known international standards vary when performed in distinguished centers (3,5). The important point is to define its degree of variation and an acceptable confidence limit.

The final part corresponds to in vivo studies. Four hemophilia A patients have received different batches of the local therapeutic concentrates (8). The recovery was assessed according to Allain et al. (9), who demonstrated that highest plasma factor VIII elevation occurs between 15-60 minutes post transfusion. Table 6 shows the in vivo recovery at 15 and 60 minutes post infusion, measured against the local concentrate standard which, in its turn is coupled to the international concentrate standard (fig. 2). The expected factor VIII rise is calculated according to the body weights as well as to the plasma volumes. In 10 of the 11 batches recovery was 100%. The lower recovery might be due to the timing of the sampling; a 30 or 45 minute samples should have been more appropriate. Alternative explanations could be an overlabeling of the potency of the product or due to the recipient himself.

From this study it is concluded that it is very important to use appropriate factor VIII:C standards for assessing both in vitro and in vivo activities of factor VIII products.

Table 6. Factor VIII:C infusion and in-vivo recovery.

Patient	Batch no.	Units inf.	15 min.	60 min.	Expected
1	83C0801 83B1501	976	0.42	0.34	0.50*/0.43**
	83B1801	632	0.32	0.36	0.32 /0.28
2	83C1601	848	0.37	0.49	0.37 /0.31
	83B2301	840	0.33	0.38	0.36 /0.31
3	83C0401	1452	0.42	0.37	0.47 /0.39
	83C0201 83C2401	1504	0.46	0.46	0.46 /0.40
4	83B1501 83B2101	1132	0.37	0.35	0.36 /0.30
	83C1001	1540	0.30	0.27	0.49/ 0.41

* calculated expected values to patient plasma volume
** calculated expected values to patient body weight

REFERENCES

1. Austen DEG, Rhymes IR, Rizza CR. Factor VIII concentrates: what the label says. Lancet, 1981;ii:1167.
2. Kasper CK. Problems with the potency of factor VIII concentrates. N Engl J Med, 1981;305:50-1.
3. Barrowcliffe TW, Curtis AD, Thomas DP. Standardization of factor VIII. IV Establishment of the 3rd international standard for factor VIII:C concentrate. Thromb Haemost, 1983;50:697-702.
4. Barrowcliffe TW, Kirkwood TBL. Principles of bioassay of haemostatic components. In: Haemostatis and Thrombosis. Bloom EL, Thomas DP, eds. Churchill Livingstone, Edinburgh. 1981:832-44.
5. Barrowcliffe TW, Tydeman MW, Kirkwood TBL, Thomas DP. Standardization of factor VIII. III. Establishment of a suitable reference plasma for factor VIII related activities. Thromb Haemost, 1983;50:690-6.

6. Godfrey R, Rhymes IL, Bidwell E, Barrowcliffe TW. The buffering of anticoagulants for blood collection. Thrombos Diathes Haemorr, 1975;34:879-82.
7. Lusher JM, Fusll FAO, Edson JR et al. North American study of factor VIII concentrate potency. Scand J Haematol, 1984;33 (suppl.40): 149-60.
8. Smit Sibinga CTh, Daenen SMG, van Imhoff GW, Maas A, Das PC. Heparin small pool high yield purified factor VIII: In vivo recovery and half-life of routinely produced freeze-dried concentrate. Thromb Haemost, 1984;51:12-5.
9. Allain JP, Verroust F, Soulier JP. In vitro and in vivo characterization of factor VIII preparations. Vox Sang, 1980;38:68-80.

THE CURRENT OF STATUS OF FIBRONECTIN IN CLINICAL MEDICAL PRACTICE

E.L. Snyder

Fibronectin is a dimeric glycoprotein with a molecular weight of 400,000 to 440,000 daltons composed of two 220,000 dalton subunit chains linked by disulfide bridges. It participates in host defenses by acting as a nonspecific opsonin, capable of removing non-bacterial debris from blood including fibrinogen/fibrin complexes, collagenous debris, denatured proteins and remnants of cellular cytoskeleton. Such debris may occur after trauma, sepsis, burn injury, or disseminated intravascular coagulation (DIC). This material may also be passively infused in blood transfusions which contain microaggregate debris.

The normal range of fibronectin is between 180 g/ml and 720 g/ml, with a mean value of 320 g/ml. Although patients with sepsis, trauma, or burns have documented deficiencies of fibronectin. the question remains as to whether a deficiency of this opsonic glycoprotein is consistently associated with disease. Further, the question of whether elevation of fibronectin levels reverse or ameliorate a disease process also remains to be evaluated. This paper will address the current clinical status of fibronectin based on published data from human studies. The major question to be addressed is whether fibronectin is, at present, therapeutically useful for treatment of human illness. To answer this question the risk:benefit ratio must be considered, as it needs to be considered prior to administration of any blood product capable of transmitting hepatitis or AIDS.

INTERACTION OF FIBRONECTIN WITH THE RES

Fibronectin has been shown to be closely involved with the reticulo-endothelial system. Macrophages can produce fibronectin (1) and mono-cytes have receptors for fibronectin on their surface as well (2). Following fibronectin attachment to monocytes, there is enhanced expression of monocyte receptors for the Fc fragment of IgG and the C3 component of complement as well as secretion of neutral proteases (2). With such enhancement of receptors, monocytes can function more efficiently (3). Pommier et al., (4) showed that fibronectin enhances monocyte phagocytosis by stimulating monocytes to ingest debris already opsonized with C3b and IgG. Fibronectin can also promote differentation of monocytes into inflammatory macrophages (5), which can clear debris and blood clots from intravascular sites thus promoting organ blood flow. Fibronectin binds to Staphylococci but not to most Gram negative organisms (6,7,8). Although binding to Staphylococcus aureus, fibro-nectin does not promote phagocytosis of bacteria by either granulocytes or monocytes (8,9). Other data, however, has shown conflicting results (10,11). Further studies are needed to fully elucidate the role of fibro-nectin in bacterial phagocytosis.

FIBRONECTIN BIOASSAY VS. IMMUNOASSAY

One area of growing interest and concern is the appropriate method to use for measuring fibronectin. Most methods in current use are immunological methods. The Laurell rocket immunoelectrophoretic technique using monospecific rabbit or goat-anti human fibronectin antibody was the method originally used in clinical studies. An immunoturbidimetric assay is also available as a commercial kit (12). Fibronectin bioassays are also in use. One is a functional assay which quantitates the uptake of a radiolabelled lipid emulsion by rat liver slices in the presence of heparin and plasma fibronectin (13). Another bioassay uses rat peritoneal macrophages while another uses human monocytes (14). Discrepancies between the immunoreactive levels of fibronectin and bioassayable fibronectin have been reported (15,16). Theories to explain this divergence have been proposed (17) and include a possible adverse effect of actin binding to fibronectin which would alter the bioassayable levels of fibronectin but not the antigenic immunoassay.

SAMPLE COLLECTION

Collection of fibronectin by percutaneous venipuncture can be difficult as many critically ill patients do not have good vascular access due to the presence of multiple indwelling catheters. Obtaining blood samples for fibronectin assay through indwelling plastic catheters could, in theory, produce artefactually lowered levels of fibronectin as these catheters are known to become partially occluded with fibrin and are usually flushed with heparin. Fibronectin is known to bind to fibrin and to be precipitable by heparin in the cold. Studies by Snyder et al. (18), however, have shown that measurements of fibronectin from samples obtained through indwelling plastic intravenous, Swan-Ganz, or arterial catheters were equivalent to those values obtained after simultaneous, percutaneous venipuncture. Bowen et al. (19) has described some variables which affect fibronectin sample collection, separation and storage.

FIBRONECTIN LEVELS IN DISEASE

The levels of fibronectin in a variety of hematologic and epithelial cell malignancies have been reported (20-22), and show wide variations in fibronectin levels. It is clear from reviewing these data that fibronectin levels must be measured in individual patients as levels fluctuate widely. Low levels of fibronectin in patients with malignancy and associated DIC have been reported by Mosher et al. (23). Fibronectin levels may be affected by treatment of the disease process as well. As reported by Brodin et al. (24), plasma fibronectin levels fell during chemotherapy for treatment of acute myeloid leukemia; Choate et al (22) reported similar findings. As the hepatocyte is felt to be the major, albeit not the only, site of fibronectin synthesis, metastatic or primary liver disease may lower fibronectin levels in patients with malignancy as well (25). Thus, evaluation of fibronectin in malignant conditions is difficult as the level of fibronectin in these patients may be altered by the presence of sepsis, DIC trauma, chemotherapy, liver involvement or other clinical variables.

Importantly, fibronectin's role in malignancy may be more global than originally thought. Perri et al. (26) showed that fibronectin may be involved with regulatory control over neoplastic proliferation. Preliminary reports showed that purified firbonectin is capable of increasing both fresh and cultured human monocyte and macrophage tumor-directed cytotoxicity. Divergence between levels of bioassayable and immunoreactive fibronectin in studies involving mouse tumors have been reported (15) and may shed doubt on the suitability of clinical studies which have monitored only immunoreactive levels of fibronectin; furhter data is needed in this area.

In studies of non-malignant disease, fibronectin concentrations were elevated in patients with acute viral hepatitis but not other types of liver disease such as alcoholic liver disease (27). Patients with other non-malignent diseases such as sepsis, trauma, or burns are discussed below.

TRANSFUSION OF FIBRONECTIN

Fibronectin is stable in whole blood, single donor plasma, fresh frozen plasma and platelet concentrates (28). The highest concentration of fibronectin is found in cryoprecipitate which has a 10 fold higher level of fibronectin than does human plasma. The level of fibronectin in various blood components is an important consideration when transfusing critically ill patients with fibronectin as a form of drug therapy. Saba et al. (29) has commented that elevated levels of fibronectin in excess of normal levels due to hyper-transfusion could result in particulate aggregation and microembolization of debris to the pulmonary or other capillary beds. Thus levels of fibronectin should be measured and found to be below the lower limit of normal (<180 μg/ml) before instituting therapy. The optimal dosage of fibronectin is unknown. Most authors transfuse cryoprecipitate prepared from 10 units of fresh frozen plasma as a single infusion (30,31,32). Frequency of fibronectin administration is not standardized either. A reasonable recommendation is to transfuse fibronectin in response to obtaining a plasma value below the lower limit of 180 μg/ml, although there is truthfully no data to support such a recommendation with any certainty. The duration of fibronectin elevation in response to infusion of cryoprecipitate is unknown and probably varies with each patient. Thus periodic measurements of plasma fibronectin levels are needed when evaluating patients being treated with this opsonic glycoprotein.

If demand for fibronectin were to increase appreciably the production of cryoprecipitate would increase perhaps at the expense of hemophiliacs and patients with von Willebrand's disease who depend on cryoprecipitate for factor VIII. Use of source plasma for production of a parenteral form of fibronectin could compete with plasma needed for production of albumin, plasma protein fraction, and gamma globulin.

In addition to the concern over sufficient amounts of plasma to meet all the demands for plasma products, the concern over the stability of purified firbonectin should be raised. Boughton et al. (33) have reported that for affinity purified firbonectin, cold storage at -20°C or heat treatment at 56°C results in loss of opsonic function probably due to a conformational change in the protein structure. With this purified form of fibronectin appearing unstable for long term storage, fresh frozen plasma or cryoprecipitate appears to be the best alternative for fibronectin therapy. Saba et al. (29), however, has suggested that the biological activity of fibronectin in cryoprecipitate may only remain intact for 4 months. More data on the stability of parenteral fibronectin preparations as well as on fibronectin stored as frozen plasma or cryoprecipitate are needed. The need for such studies is clearly predicated on the proof that fibronectin will be clinical useful, an area itself in need of further investigation.

HUMAN CLINICAL TRIALS

Several publications have reviewed the literature involving the usefulness of fibronectin (29,34,35,36). Fibronectin administered in uncontrolled studies has been associated with clinical improvement (31,37,38). Until recently no studies had confirmed that it was the fibronectin per se in cryoprecipitate which was responsible for the improvement in reticuloendothelial cell function. A controlled study by Saba et al. (16) recently showed an improvement in fibronectin levels and reticuloendothelial cell function with cryoprecipitate but not cryoprecipitate-extracted (fibronectin depleted) plasma. This study also showed, as mentioned above, that the bioassayable levels of fibronectin are not as well maintained as are the values for the immunoreactive antigenic assays.

Although fibronectin levels have been shown to fall after cardiopulmonary bypass surgery (18,39) these decreases were transient. Snyder et al. (18) showed that levels of fibronectin <180 μg/ml were only seen in postoperative patients who were critically ill. Prophylactic administration of fibronectin was unnecessary in these studies. The results of these two studies has provided useful data on the types of patients who might require fibronectin therapy. Clearly, the clinical sequelae from major surgery has not been shown to consistently require fibronectin supplementation. A major question concerns the use of fibronectin to predict the onset of sepsis (40,41). Most studies have shown that fibronectin is not predictive of sepsis (18,42,43) or that if it is associated with sepsis, the temporal relationship is too close to permit significant clinical advantage over the standard practice of close clinical monitoring. Richards et al. (44) studied levels of fibronectin in 16 patients with intra-abdominal infection. The conclusion of their study was that they could not accurately predict on the basis of fibronectin levels which of the 16 patients were likely to develop multiple organ failure.

Firbonectin administration may not be the complete answer to the problem of reticuloendothelial cell dysfunction. Lanser et al. (45) showed that the abnormal changes in RES function in burn-injured rats were not reversed by administration of fibronectin. Thus RES function may rely on factors other than just replacement of fibronectin. Rubli et al. (46) showed that decreasing levels of fibronectin were seen in septic patients but that this decline was not prognostic of mortality and was part of a general decline in plasma proteins seen in these acutely septic patients. Monitoring fibronectin levels in these patients was not predictive of clinical course either.

CONCLUSIONS

The conlcusions from this brief review of the literature are:
1. Fibronectin deficiency is not consistently associated with organ failure but may be seen in patients with critical illness accompanied by sepsis and DIC.
2. There are insufficient numbers of well controlled clinical studies to determine if elevation of fibronectin levels will reverse or ameliorate a disease process.

3. Changes in immunoassayable fibronectin do not always correspond to changes in bioassayable fibronectin.
4. There are, currently, no firm guidelines for determining treatment dose, frequency of administration or form of therapy i.e., cryoprecipitate vs a parenteral preparation.
5. Since there are no controlled studies which clearly show a benefit from fibronectin administration, there are no specific patients groups for whom fibronectin therapy can be recommended.
6. Although septic patients have lower levels of fibronectin than non-septic patients, the fall in levels of fibronectin has not been shown to be a better predictor of morbidity or mortality than close clinical observation.
7. Blinded controlled trials in humans are needed to show that fibronectin is a useful therapeutic modality.

Although fibronectin may prove to be useful for some critically ill patients it is unlikely to become the general panacea that was once hoped for (35). Its role in clinical medicine remains to be defined.

REFERENCES

1. Alitalo K, Hovi T, Vaheri A. Fibronectin is produced by human macrophages. J Exp Med 1980;151:602-13.
2. Bevilacqua Mp, Amrani D, Mosesson MW, Bianco C. Receptors for cold insoluble globulin (plasma fibronectin) on human monocytes. J Exp Med 1981;153:42-60.
3. Postlethwaite AE, Keski-Oja J, Balian G, Kang A. Induction of fibroblast chemotaxis by fibronectin. Localization of the chemotactic region to a 140,000 molecular weight non-gelatin-binding fragment. J Exp Med 1981;153:494-9.
4. Pommier CG, Inada S, Fries LF, Takahashi T, Frank MM, Brown EJ. Plasma fibronectin enhances phagocytosis of opsonized particles by human peripheral blood monocytes. J Exp Med 1983;157:1844-54.
5. Bianco C. Fibrin, fibronectin and macrophages. Ann Ny Acad Sci 1983;408:602-9.
6. Mosher DF, Proctor RA. Binding and factor XIIIa-mediated cross-linking of a 27 kilodalton fragment of fibronectin to Staphylococcus aureus. Science 1980;209:927-9.
7. Kuusela P. Fibronectin binds to Staphylococcus aureus. Nature 1978;276:718-20.
8. Van de Water L, Destree AT, Hynes RO. Fibronectin binds to some bacteria but does not promote their uptake by phagocytic cells. Science 1983;220:201-4.
9. Proctor RA, Prendergast E, Mosher DF. Fibronectin mediated attachment of Staphylococcus aureus to human neutrophils. Blood 1982;59:681-7.
10. Lanser ME, Saba TM. Opsonic fibronectin is necessary for optimal serum-mediated phagocytosis of Staphylococcus aureus by human neutrophils. Adv Shock Res 1982;8:111.
11. Lanser ME, Saba TM. Fibronectin as a co-factor necessary for optimal granulocyte phagocytosis of Staphylococcus aureus. J Reticuloendothel Soc 1981;30:415-24.
12. Saba TM, Albert WH, Blumenstock FA, Evanega G, Staehler F, Cho E. Evaluation of rapid immunoturbidimetric assay for opsonic fibronectin in surgical and trauma patients. J Lab Clin Med 1981; 98:482-91.

13. Blumenstock FA, Saba TM, Weber P, Laffin R. Biochemical and immunological characterization of human opsonic α_2 SB glycoprotein: its identity with cold-insoluble globulin. J Biol Chem 1978;253: 4287-91.
14. Blumenstock FA, Saba TM, Roccario E, Cho E, Kaplan JE. Opsonic fibronectin after trauma and particle injection determined by a peritoneal macrophage monolayer assay. J Reticuloendothel Soc 1981;30:61-71.
15. Saba TM, Gregory TJ, Blumenstock FA. Circulating immunoreactive and bioassayable opsonic plasma fibronectin during experimental tumor growth. Br J Cancer 1980;41:956-65.
16. Saba TM, Blumenstock FA, Shah DM, et al. Reversal of fibronectin and opsonic deficiency in patients. Ann Surg 1984;199:87-96.
17. Dillon BC, Estes JE, Saba TM, et al. Actin-induced reticuloendothelial phagocytic depression as mediated by its interaction with fibronectin. Experimental Pathol 1983;38:208-23.
18. Snyder E, Barash P. Mosher DF, Walter SD. Plasma fibronectin level and clinical status in cardiac surgery patients. J Lab Clin Med 1983;102:881-9.
19. Bowen M, Muller T. Influence of sample preparation on estimates of blood fibronectin concentration. J Clin Pathol 1981;36:233-5.
20. Boughton BJ, Simpson A. Plasma fibronectin in acute leukemia. Brit J Haematol 1982;51:487-91.
21. Norfolk DR, Bowen M, Roberts BE, Child JA. Plasma fibronectin in myeloproliferative disorders and chronic granulocytic leukaemia. Brit J Haematol 1983;55:319-24.
22. Choate JJ, Mosher DF. Fibronectin concentration in plasma of patients with breast cancer, colon cancer and acute leukemia. Cancer 1983;51:1142-7.
23. Mosher DF, Williams EM. Fibronectin concentration is decreased in plasma of severely ill patients with disseminated intravascular coagulation. J Lab Clin Med 1978;91:729-35.
24. Brodin B, Lieden G, Malm C, Vikrot O. Plasma fibronectin deficiency during chemotherapy of acute myeloid leukemia. Scan J Haem 1983;30:247-9.
25. Owens MR, Cimino CD. Synthesis of fibronectin by the isolated perfused rat liver. Blood 1982;59:1305-9.
26. Perri RT, Kay NE, McCarthy J, Vessella RL, Jacobs HS, Furcht LT. Fibronectin enhances in vitro monocyte-macrophage-mediated tumoricidal activity. Blood 1982;60:430-5.
27. Gluud C, Dejgaard A, Clemmensen I. Plasma fibronectin concentrations in patients with liver diseases. Scand J Clin Lab Invest 1983;43:533-7.
28. Snyder EL, Ferri PM, Mosher DF. Fibronectin in liquid and frozen stored blood components. Transfusion 1984;24:53-6.
29. Saba TM. Reversal of plasma Fn deficiency in septic-injured patients by cryoprecipitate infusion. In: Massive Transfusion in Surgery and Trauma. Collins JA, Murawski K, Shafer AW eds. New York, A.R. Liss 1982:129-150.
30. Annest SJ, Scovill WA, Blumenstock FA, et al. Increased creatinine clearance following cryoprecipitate infusion in trauma and surgical patients with decreased renal function. J Trauma 1980;20:726-32.
31. Scovill WA, Saba TM, Blumenstock FA, et al. Opsonic α_2 surface binding glycoprotein therapy during sepsis. Ann Surg 1978;188: 521-9.

32. Scovill WA, Annest SJ, Saba TM, et al. Cardiopulmonary hemodynamics after opsonic α-2 surface binding glycoprotein therapy in injured patients. Surgery 1979;86:284-93.

33. Boughton BJ, Simpson A, Wharton C. Conformational charges and loss of opsonic function in frozen or heat-treated plasma fibronectin. Vox Sang 1984;46:254-9.

34. Mosher DF. Fibronectin. Prog Hemostasis and Thrombosis 1980;5: 111-51.

35. Mosher DF, Grossman JE. Clinical use of fibronectin. La Ricerca Clin Lab 1983;13:43-54.

36. Furcht L. Structure and function of the adhesive glycoprotein fibronectin. Modern Cell Biol 1983;1:53-117.

37. Saba TM. Prevention of liver reticuloendothelial systemic host defense failure after surgery by intravenous opsonic glycoprotein therapy. Ann Surg 1978;188:142-52.

38. Saba TM, Blumenstock FA, Scovill WA, Bernard H. Cryoprecipitate reversal of opsonic α_2 surface binding glycoprotein deficiency in septic surgical and trauma patients. Science 1978;201:622-4.

39. Gandhi JG, Vander Salm T, Szymanski IO. Effect of cardiopulmonary bypass on plasma fibronectin, IgG and C3. Transfusion 1983;23:476-9.

40. Brodin B, Berghem L, Friberg-Nielson S, Nordstrom H, Schildt B. Fibronectin in the treatment of septicemia — a preliminary report. In: 7th World Congress of Anesthesiology Hamburg, Excerpta Medica 1980:504-5.

41. Lanser ME, Saba TM, Scovill WA. Opsonic glycoprotein (plasma fibronectin) levels after burn injury. Relationship to extent of burn and development of sepsis. Ann Surg 1980;192:776-82.

42. Dietch EA, Gelder F, McDonald JC. The relationship between CIg depletion and peripheral neutrophil function in rabbits and man. J Trauma 1982;22:469-75.

43. Dietch EA, Gelder F, McDonald JC. Sequential prospective analysis of the nonspecific host defense system after thermal injury. Arch Surg 1984;119:83-9.

44. Richards WO, Scovill WA, Baekhyo S. Opsonic fibronectin deficiency in patients with intra-abdominal infection. Surgery 1983;94:210-7.

45. Lanser ME, Saba TM. Correction of serum opsonic defects after burn and sepsis by opsonic fibronectin administration. Arch Surg 1983;118:338-42.

46. Rubli E, Bussard S, Frei E, Lundsgaard-Hansen P. Pappova E. Plasma fibronectin and associated variables in surgical intensive care patients. Ann Surg 1983;197:310-7.

INTRAVENOUS USE OF GAMMAGLOBULIN IN 1984

J.B. Bussel

Intravenous use of gammaglobulin therapy has been proven to be a major advance over intramuscular therapy in certain settings. This difference is due completely to consideration of dosage; the antibodies themselves are identical and come from identical sources of plasma and Cohn fractions. This increased dosage has expanded potential for antibody replacement and also has led to new application to the treatment of autoimmune disease.

Previous usage of intramuscular gammaglobulin as replacement therapy of hypogammaglobulinemia had been limited by the volume of the 16% gammaglobulin preparation possible per injection and the patient's ability to tolerate a number of injections. One trial carried out in the 1960's showed that 25 mg/kg/week of IM gammaglobulin was equivalent in clinical effect to 50 mg/kg/week and since that time the generally accepted dosage of gammaglobulin for replacement therapy has been 25 mg/kg/week usually given as 2 large injections (one in each buttock) every 2 weeks (1). Adults, even with 2 x 5 ml injections, fall short of 25 mg/kg/week and such injections are generally painful. In addition a percentage of the administered gammaglobulin may be catabolized by proteolytic enzymes at the site of injection. This therefore also limits the dosage and several days are required for absorbtion of the injected gammaglobulin so that peak blood levels are not attained until 3 to 7 days after injection.

In contrast, with the currently available preparations of gammaglobulin suitable for intravenous use, the dosage can be chosen by the treating physician and set at any suitable level. The infused material is all available for physiological usage to the patient and peak blood levels occur immediately upon infusion. The major question with the intravenous preparations has been the delivery of unmodified fully functional immunoglobulin that will be safe and not lead to reactions caused by intravenous infusion of IgG aggregates. While the exact pathophysiology of adverse reactions to immunoglobulin administration (whether IV or IM) remains poorly understood, early studies of intravenous infusion of the intramuscular preparations led to severe anaphyllactoid reactions that appeared to be due to the IgG aggregates in the preparations and their capability to spontaneously activate the complement (2). Therefore, preparation of immunoglobulin concentrates suitable for intravenous usage has involved removal of existing IgG aggregates (created by the plasma fractionation procedure) and preventing formation of new aggregates. The first generation of such preparations centered around enzymatic digestion of the immunoglobulin, usually with plasmin, in order to eliminate the ability of the immunoglobulin molecules to activate complement. Subsequently it was discovered that the antibody molecules were so damaged that their functions were often interfered with and the half lives considerably shortened. The second generation of products included milder modification of the immunoglobulin molecule utilizing interruption of disulfide bridges in the Fc portion of the molecule, again with the intent to interfere with complement activation and aggregation if IgG monomers. However the loss of integrity of the Fc region in these preparations, (in the absence of comparative controlled trials) has

resulted in a clinical impression that the unmodified preparations currently undergoing trials are likely to be superior. It appears at present
that isolated fully functional immunoglobulin molecules can be delivered
to almost all patients for whom such treatment is desired safely and at
high dose.

Who are the patients for whom such treatment is desireable? The first
and most obvious group includes those patients who are antibody deficient
and in turn the most obvious group of these patients are those who are
congenitally hypogammaglobulinemic. Several published trials of IVGG
administration in congenitally hypogammaglobulinemic patients have been
performed. One trial utilizing an alkylated and reduced preparation of
IVGG at equivalent dosage to IMGG showed no advantage of IVGG (3);
a second trial of the same preparation utilizing 0 mg/kg/week IV versus
25 mg/kg/week IM showed a clear advantage of IV over the IM treatment
(4). Recently a controlled trial in 21 patients of one year of IMGG
20 mg/kg/week compared to one year of IVGG at 100 mg/kg/week using
a pH4 treated preparation showed dramatic reductions (greater than 50%)
in days sick and days of antibiotic usage even in there chronically ill
patients (5). All subtypes of specific illness were improved except for
gastrointestinal disease. Concomitant with the clinical improvements was
an average elevation of the trough IgG levels of 250 mg/dl above the
trough levels seen with the lower level of the normal range. A specially
selected group of chronically ill hypogammaglobulinemic patients with
sinopulmonary disease were treated at the high dose of 150 mg/kg/week
with the pH4 preparation. The majority ultimately had significant clinical
improvement and were able to eventually discontinue their continuous
antibiotic usage. However, both clinical improvement and stable trough
IgG levels (in the middle of the normal range) were only attained after
more than one year of therapy (6). In addition preliminary results
suggest that salivary IgG was only detectable after one year of this
very high dose therapy. While not many controlled trials have been
completed, it appears at present that the higher dosage of gammaglobulin
which can be delivered by the intravenous route will benefit at least
some patients. The exact dosage required is uncertain as is the best
"philosophy" of treatment. Some clinicians currently advocate the use of
IVGG (and higher serum IgG levels) only for the persistently sick
patients; other feel that effective prophylaxis requires a high dose of
IVGG to be delivered routinely to all patients. The role of IVGG therapy
in regard to the T-cell defects seen in approximately half such patients
is uncertain as is the role of IVGG replacement in possible prophylaxis
of gastrointestinal malignancies and lymphomas which develop with increased frequency in these patients. The likely minimum dosage would
be 50 mg/kg/week and the interval every 3 or 4 weeks but further
studies are required in order to be more definitive.

The usage of IVGG as detailed above has been widely generalized to
other settings of hypogammaglobulinemia although few to no results of
clinical trials are yet available. The areas in which IVGG has been most
frequently used include hypogammaglobulinemia of prematurity and
advanced stages of CLL. Studies reflecting safety and likely efficacy of
IVGG in prematures have been published (7) and premature infants
certainly are a hypogammaglobulinemic group with a high incidence of
sepsis. Similarly most patients with CLL have a B-cell malignancy and,
especially in the advanced stages and after several years have passed,
these patients are often hypogammaglobulinemic. Furhtermore, these
patients are often troubled by infections and their major complications
are bleeding and infections (due to the relatively indolent nature of the
leukemia). Other diseases associated with hypogammaglobulinemia include

Wiskott Aldrich syndrome and IgA-IgG$_2$ deficiency. The Wiskott Aldrich syndrome may include hypercatabolism of immunoglobulin and therefore may require higher dosage of immunoglobulin more frequently although little data in this regard is available. IgA-IgG$_2$ deficient patients illustrate the category of patients who are partially hypogammaglobulinemic and therefore may be at risk to make antibody to the infused gammaglobulin; problems of this type have not been reported. States of "acquired" antibody deficiency where IVGG might be beneficial include "contaminated" abdominal surgery, severe trauma, and burns. These settings are united by a decrease in gammaglobulin level and a high incidence of infection. Preliminary results of the usage of IVGG in surgical patients and in trauma patients suggest benefit. Patients with serious burns and with major operations decrease their gammaglobulin levels and patients with severe trauma often are on respirators which gives them a proclivity to infection. Patients with multiple myeloma also are antibody deficient and hypercatabolize IgG due to their elevated immunoglobulin level; consequently they may be particularly difficult to treat (8).

Another type of usage involves prophylaxis or treatment of viral infections in certain settings. Immunosuppressed patients with varicella zoster infections have recently been successfully treated with IVGG (9). Animal work and preliminary results of human studies imply that respiratory syncytial virus infections also can be treated with IVGG, albeit at higher dosage. The optimum situation to use IVGG for prophylaxis of a viral infection appears to be the prevention of cytomegalovirus pneumonitis after bone marrow transplantation. Again preliminary data suggest that IVGG may have a role (10) but controlled trials are needed.

Other usage of IVGG in antibody deficiency is still entirely speculative. Certain patients with IgG subclass deficiency and/or an inability to make specific antibodies may also benefit from IVGG. Other patients may have their primary antibody response temporarily impaired, such as during induction chemotherapy of leukemia, and thereby benefit from IVGG.

A final usage of IVGG involves the recent speculation about possibility of anti-idiotypic immune suppression (11). Certain persistent or recurrent infections may occur because the anti-idiotype predominates and completely suppresses production of the primary antibody. IVGG would provide the primary antibody so that the infection could be cleared or prevented.

In summary patients with congenital hypogammaglobulinemia are likely to benefit from the higher doses of gammaglobulin replacement available by the intravenous route. Guidelines would include the use of an unmodified gammaglobulin preparation if available, a suggested dose of 100 mg/kg/week for therapy and/or prophylaxis of bacterial infections, and the assessment of specific titers within the preparation if these are important. For example, recent work has demonstrated a very low titer of anti-urea plasma antibody in the preparations and therefore treatment of these infections is likely to be ineffective (12). In a given setting i.e. post bone marrow transplant it may be desirable to insure a high titer against a specific organism with a hyperimmune preparation. However in any clinical setting the use of a broad spectrum preparation of antibodies has merit over a monoclonal antibody infusion.

The usage of IVGG in autoimmune disease has proven to be an unexpected benefit of the ability to deliver high dosage. The original work in this field was the report in 1981 by Imbach et al. of the efficacy of 2 gm/kg of IVGG in the treatment of idiopathic thrombocytopenic purpura (13). While the exact clinical role has been extensively analyzed the mechanism of action is important to discuss in relationship to other potential uses.

The most clearcut effect of IVGG in ITP is RES Fc receptor blockade (14). This effect presumably lengthens antibody coated platelet survival leading to a higher platelet count. Antibody coated red cell clearance studies suggest that this effect may last up to 4 weeks accounting for the acute increase and decrease in the platelet count. Some patients treated by IVGG appear to derive a long term benefit from therapy presumably mediated by a decrease in autoantibody synthesis. Evidence for this effect has been elusive. Recent investigation in ITP suggests that many patients may be IgG subclass deficient (especially IgG_2) (15) and IVGG may restore normal feedback control of autoantibody synthesis as seen in several patients (16). However, platelet antibody levels do not clearly decrease in treated patients even with good increases in the platelet count.

The possibility of suppression of anti-platelet antibody synthesis led to treatment of other autoantibody mediated diseases where RES blockade is not involved. One report shows that all 5 patients with SLE-ITP had decreases in autoantibody (anti thyroid, anti DNA) titers concomitant with IVGG therapy (17). Similarly some patients with myasthenia gravis appear to benefit from IVGG. Finally one congenital hemophiliac with an inhibitor to factor IX and several patients with acquired autoantibodies to factor VIII have all responded well to IVGG therapy. The implications in the factor IX patient was that the IVGG induced the development of an anti-idiotypic antibody (18). However, the overall effects of using IVGG in these patients have proven disappointing and relatively few patients appear to have clearcut response. It is possible that higher doses i.e. 5 gm/kg of IVGG would have sufficient effect to make the response more generalized or, alternatively that only certain patients are capable of responding to IVGG. Much further study is required if IVGG is to be a generally usefull therapy in autoimmune diseases.

In summary IVGG has been a significant therapeutic advance for many diseases. A major advantage, and the reason that it has been so extensively utilized, is its almost complete lack of toxicity. Various studies have shown no interference in the ability to make antibodies or in various cell mediated immune functions. No longterm deterioration of immune responsiveness has been seen and no cases of hepatitis of AIDS transmission reported. One patient has been reported who developed candida sepsis after IVGG usage possible because of the RES blockade. Reactions associated with administration have not been a serious problem when the appropriate precautions are taken. At this time it appears that IVGG will have multiple uses in the role of antibody replacement therapy but its use in autoimmune disease is currently limited to certain cases of the immune cytopenias.

REFERENCES

1. Hill LE, Mollison PL. Conclusions. In: Hypogammaglobulinemia. United Kingdom Medical Research Council; MRC Special Report Series, no. 310,1971.
2. Barandun S, Kistler P, Jeunet F, Isliker H. Intravenous administration of human gammaglobulin. Vox Sang 1962;7:157-62.
3. Ammann AJ, Ashman RF, Buckley RH et al. Use of intravenous gammaglobulin in antibody immunodeficiency: results of a multicenter controlled trial. Clin Immunol Immunopathol. 1982;22:60-7.

4. Nolte MT, Pirofsky B, Gerritz GA, Golding B. Intravenous immuno-globulin therapy of antibody deficiency. Clin exp Immunol 1979; 36:237-43.
5. Cunningham-Rundles C, Siegal FP, Smithwick EM et al. Efficacy of intravenous immunoglobulin in primary humoral immunodeficiency disease. Ann of Intern Med 1984;101:435-9.
6. Gelfand E. Treatment of chronic infections in hypogammaglobuline-mia with very high dose intravenous gammaglobulin. In: Intravenous immunoglobulin in immunodeficiency syndromes and in ITP. Ed: Webster ADB, and Waters AH. Int Congress and Symposium Series. Pub: Roy Soc Med, London; 1985.
7. Von Muralt G, Sidiropoulos D. Le traitement substitutif par les immunoglobulines en neonatologie. la Presse Med 1983;12:2595-602.
8. Gordon DS, Hearn EB, Spira TJ, Reimer CB, Phillips DJ, Schable C. Phase I study of intravenous gammaglobulin in multiple myeloma Am J Med 1984;76:111-6.
9. Sulliser JM, Imbach P, Barandun S, et al. Varicella and herpes zoster in immunosuppressed children: preliminary results of treatment with intravenous immunoglobulin. Helv Pediatr Acta 1984; 39:63-70.
10. Condie RM, O'Reilly RJ. Prevention of cytomegalovirus infection by prophylaxis with an intravenous, hyperimmune, native, unmodified cytomegalovirus globulin. Am J Med 1984;76:134-41.
11. Nydegger UE, Blaser K, Hässig A. Antiidiotypic immunosuppression and its treatment with human immunoglobulin preparations. Vox Sang 1984;47:92-5.
12. Lever AML. The role of opsonic antibody in host defence. In: Intra-venous immunoglobulin in immunodeficiency syndromes and in ITP. ED: Webster ADB, and Waters AH. Int Congress and Symposium Series. Roy Soc Med, London; 1985.
13. Imbach P, d'Apuzzi V, Hirt A, et al. High-dose intravenous gamma-globulin for idiopathic thrombocytopenic purpura in childhood. Lancet. 1981;i:1228.
14. Bussel JB, Imberly RP, Inman RD, et al. Intravenous gamma-globulin treatment of chronic idiopathic thrombocytopenic purpura. Blood 1983;62:480-6.
15. Bussel J, Morell A, Porges A, et al. Selective IgG_2 deficiency in patients with ITP. Abstract. ASH, 1984.
16. Bussel J, Porges A, Pahwa S, et al. Intravenous gammaglobulin in ITP: Effect on antibody synthesis. Abstract. ASH, 1983.
17. Tsubakio T, Kurata Y, Katagiri S, et al. Alteration of T cell subsets and immunoglobulin synthesis in vitro during high dose gamma-globulin therapy in patients with idiopathic thrombocytopenic purpura. Clin exp Immunol 1983;53:697-702.
18. Nilsson IM, Sundqvist SB. Suppression of secondary antibody response by intravenous immunoglobulin and development of tolerance in a patient with haemophilia B and antibodies. Scand J Haematol 1984;33:203-6.

DISCUSSION

Moderators: F. Peetoom, C.Th. Smit Sibinga

W.G. van Aken:

Dr. Bussel, I have two questions related to the data you presented on the usage of intravenous immunoglobulins for immune-deficiency patients. You mentioned that although the number of infections decreased, the number of hospital days increased. I would like to know if there was a specific reason for that discrepancy.

J.B. Bussel:

That was largely due to one patient who had a 28-day hospitalisation for pneumonia relatively early in the year. So, since the numbers were so small, I did not comment on it, but I appreciate your bringing it up.

W.G. van Aken:

My second question is related to the list of immuno-deficiencies which you thought were indications for the administration of gammaglobulin. The last one was the acquired immuno-deficiency syndrome. Is there evidence at present that these patients benefit from gammaglobulin?

J.B. Bussel:

I mentioned briefly about children, but I think that in adults there is no evidence at all that there is any specific effect. However, I think it is becoming known through the work of Dr. Fauci (1) and others that there is a lot of non-specific antibody being produced, and that AIDS perhaps is a state in which specific antibody exists. More and more, at least in the United States, people are using intravenous gammaglobulins in an attempt to provide the normal spectrum of antibodies that perhaps some of these patients lack; though they are clearly not going to help against Pneumocystis carinii or other opportunistic infections, which require intact cellular immunity to resist.

W.G. van Aken:

Do we already know what the effect is?

J.B. Bussel:

I do not know of any controlled trials. I believe that they are either being started or carried out now. In treating children, the clinicians feel

1. Lane HC, Masur H, Edgar LC, Whalen G, Rook AH, Fauci AS. Abnormalities of B-cell activation and immunoregulation in patients with the acquired immunodeficiency syndrome. N Eng J Med 1984; 309:453-8.

very strongly that they are a big help. I should add that the treatment is very low-dose with gradual build up, due to the large level of circulating complexes and the fact that — perhaps due to the immune complexes more reactions have been seen. But they feel that it significantly cuts down on infections in the children.

W.G. van Aken:

My final question is related to the administration of intravenous gammaglobulin in patients with ITP. What do you see, at present, as the indication for intravenous gammaglobulin in ITP patients? Would you advocate administering intravenous gammaglobulin very early in the treatment of chronic ITP? Would you prefer to administer it before performing a splenectomy? Before giving prednisolone? Before giving Vincristin? What should be the sequence? First splenectomy and later on intravenous gammaglobulin? What is your present position?

J.B. Bussel:

I believe you are alluding to Dr. Newland's (2) work about the idea of giving intravenous gammaglobulin to an adult at least at the time of splenectomy to ensure that the splenectomy will lead to remission. I do not know if that is founded or not, but it certainly seems like a potentially very interesting area. In an article published in "Blut" in August (3) it has been implied that the authors were setting up a controlled trial, but I do not know if that is the case or not.

In an adult, I personally would do splenectomy first, perhaps with gammaglobulin. Then, if the patient requires further therapy and could not be managed on relatively low doses of alternate prednisone and if cost was no object — and this is usually the big problem with this treatment — I would try intravenous gammaglobulin therapy for at least three to six months in the responding patients. We have seen a few patients who, during that process, will improve gradually. In children, essentially all chronic patients should try it. I think there may be a role in acute patients, again cost being perhaps the limiting issue.

W.G. van Aken:

So in brief, you advocate that chronic administration of intravenous gammaglobulin in ITP patients should be attempted. Not just a short course, bur for many weeks or even months.

J.B. Bussel:

Yes, Ideally, having to administer it only once every two to three weeks.

2. Newland AC, Treleaven JG, Minchinton RM, Water AH. High-dose intravenous IgG in adults with autoimmune thrombocytopenia. Lancet 1983;i:84-7.
3. Lang JM, Varadji A, Giron C, Bergerac JP, Oberling F. High-dose intravenous IgG for chronic idiopathic thrombocytopenic purpura in adults. Blut 1984;49:95-9.

K. Wallevik (Århus):

Some of us came here to get information on whether we can increase the yield in our FVIII production by using heparin as a stabiliser. We have only had small, scattered information on that subject. I know about the Groningen results (4,5) and I wonder whether others have tried to collect in heparin, and what are the results? We have tried it in Århus and compared our cryoprecipitate from blood collected in CPD with the cryoprecipitate from blood collected in heparin. We have an increase in the yield from about 35% in the CPD to about 50% in the complete parallel production in heparin.

I.M. Nilsson:

In Sweden, we are working with this problem, especially Dr. Mikealsson here. I will put the question to her.

M.E. Mikaelsson (Stockholm):

We have studied calcium stabilisation of FVIII for several years now (6). We have mainly used recalcification of CPD plasma instead of collecting in heparin. We add heparin and calcium chloride after the separation of the red cells. In this way we have managed to increase the yield by about 50% in a small scale preparation of a lyophilised intermediate purity cryoprecipitate.

S. Seidl:

I will make one small comment. This question of collecting blood in heparin instead of CPD or ACD is a very important one and has been discussed among blood bankers on several occasions. It has been nicely shown by the Groningen group that you can store these red cells when you add later on CPD anticoagulant (7). However, in spite of these data, it unfortunately is not virtually used. This is a problem which should be discussed again by all blood bankers concerned with the production of high-yield FVIII preparations. We should always put forward those questions when blood bankers are present.

C.Th. Smit Sibinga:

There has been much caution shown by Dr. Snyder about the initial storm of enthusiasm in the use of fibronectin or fibronectin-rich materials in a certain number of clinical situations. I think this point was very

4. Smit Sibinga CTh, Welbergen H, Das PC, Griffin B. High-yield method of production of freeze-dried factor VIII by blood banks. Lancet 1981;ii:449-50.
5. Smit Sibinga CTh, Das PC. Heparin and factor VIII. Scand J Haemat 1984;33 (suppl 40):111-22.
6. Mikaelsson ME, Forsman N, Oswaldsson UM. Human factor VIII: A calcium-linked protein complex. Blood 1983;62:1006-15.
7. De Jonge J, Smit Sibinga CTh, Das PC. Metabolic aspects and viability of heparin/ CPDA-1 stored red cell concentrate as a by-product of a high-yield factor VIII production method. Haemostatis 1983;13:214-8.

well brought to our notice that there is no real evidence at the moment that fibronectin really contributes to a quicker recovery and a better stabilisation of immune status of patients under severe stress, with burns, or other of these conditions. I wonder what impact that eventually might have on the efforst of certain fractionation centres in trying to purify fibronectin. Dr. Smith, could you comment on that?

J.K. Smith:

I think the situation may even be somewhat worse than Dr. Snyder has painted. This is one fractionator's point of view, I think in common with many other fractionators. Several years ago, we started to prepare fibronectin in self defense, in case the demand for fibronectin, either as fresh frozen plasma or as cryoprecipitate, would interfere too much with our FVIII supply. Like many others, we rather rapidly prepared a fibronectin concentrate which did not interfere with FVIII supplies. However, that was two years ago. The problems we have are twofold, relating to the fragmentation problem and the assay problem. They are intertwined. Now we are told that we can see fragmentation of the fibronectin molecule, as soon as or even earlier than cryoprecipitate is prepared. This means that perhaps we may be retaining the gelatin binding functions but not other important functions of the fibronectin molecule. One of our colleagues goes even further and says that fragmented firbonectin may be worse than no fibronectin at all, in that it may successfully bind the target particle but decline to opsonize it. So, we are uncertain about the clinical application and are therefore reluctant to go forward into clinical trial preparations.

The other obstacle relates to the same thing: Which assay method do you believe? So, until we have a clear statement from the interested clinicians, which assay they will believe in, i.e. which function of fibronectin they wish to have determined, we cannot match their demands with a preparation suitable for clinical use, although we are otherwise in a position to provide fibronectin quite cheaply and without interfering with FVIII.

C.Th. Smit Sibinga:

I sense from your comment and from the opening statement of Dr. Snyder that we have to reconsider which product is a contaminant of which. Now that there is not really so much need for fibronectin, I tend to stick to the statement I made: Fibronectin is more a contaminant of the FVIII production rather than the reverse. Speaking about the FVIII concentrates as these have been very eloquently tested and evaluated by Prof. Nilsson, I would like to ask a question. You showed that there is basically not much difference in recovery and in half-life no matter which product you use. In relation to the quality (in terms of specific activities) will there be a tendency in the future to go back to intermediate type of purities which do not differ that much in specific activity, compared to the high purities; or do you think there will be a tendency to go further for high-purity concentrates?

I.M. Nilsson:

I would say so, at least in Sweden. We use more and more high-purity concentrates, because it is a good concentrate and it is easy to administer to the patient for home-treatment. It is convenient for us to have a highly active concentrate in connection with major operations and for treatment of patients with inhibitors.

C.Th. Smit Sibinga:

On the other hand, we know that the more effort you put into purification the more losses you have.

I.M. Nilsson

Yes, in Sweden — as you have heard — we are working very hard to increase the yield of FVIII:C by using first DDAVP to the donors and, as Dr. Mikaelsson suggested, using recalcified and heparinized plasma.

E.L. Snyder:

Dr. Bussel, we have had occasion to attempt to use intravenous gammaglobulin, in desperation, for patients with platelet allo-antibodies. There have been two publications (8,9) recently in the American Journal of Medicine from a symposium, one of which showed a reasonable response in refractory patients after one dose of intravenous gammaglobulin. Another paper shows a rise which was not sustained. We have had conflicting results. I was wondering if you could give us some information on your experience of the use of IV-gammaglobulin for platelet allo-immunisation?

J.B. Bussel:

I do not have a great deal of personal experience, but there is also a publication in "Blood" from Schiffer et al. (10) who found absolutely no response in random donor and partially HLA-matched platelet transfusions in allo-immunised patients. I am not exactly sure why there is such a difference between ITP and allo-immune sensitization. Perhaps it is a higher level of antibody on the platelet. I consider it to be a strong evidence for the fact that RHS blockade is not the only effect of the intravenous gammaglobulin treatment.

H.D. Hory (Dreieich):

Dr. Kernoff, what kind of viruses can be transmitted by porcine FVIII. I am not a veterinarian, so I have no idea about that.

8. Junghans RP, Ahn YS. High-dose intravenous gamma globulin to suppress alloimmune destruction of donor platelets. Am J Med 1984; 76(2A):204-9.
9. Kekomäki R, Efenbein G, Gardner R, Graham-Pole J, Mehta P, Gross S. Improved response of patients refractory to random-donor platelet transfusions by intravenous gamma globulin. Am J Med 1984;76(3A):199-204.
10. Schiffer CA, Hogge DE, Aisner J, Dutcher JP, Lee EJ, Papenberg D. High-dose intravenous gammaglobulin in alloimmunized platelet transfusion recipients. Blood 1984;64:937-40.

A question to Dr. Bussel, the IVIgG preparations which were used in all the trials, I think, were produced by the Cohn method. What about the new method with the column chromatography?

J.B. Bussel:

I have no experience with the column method.

P.B.A. Kernoff:

I am no expert in that field either. But I can say that we have been to veterinarians at the London Zoo, and also to various people at the Ministry of Agriculture who are responsible for the regulations concerning importation of animal products and conditions under which products are made from animals. All these people think the risks of transmission of viruses which could infect humans must be extremely low. Last year, somebody made the suggestion that AIDS might have something to do with swine fever virus (11,12). That has absolutely been demolished. The possibility is remote.

11. Teas J. Could AIDS agent be a new variant of African swine fever virus? Lancet 1983;i:923.
12. Colaert J, Desmijter J, Goudsmit J, Clumeck N, Terpstra C. African swine fever virus antibody not found in AIDS patients. Lancet 1983; i:1098.